COVID AND CUSTOM IN RURAL SOUTH AFRICA

/ AFRICAN
/ ARGUMENTS

African Arguments is a series of short books about contemporary Africa and the critical issues and debates surrounding the continent. The books are scholarly and engaged, substantive and topical. They focus on questions of justice, rights and citizenship; politics, protests and revolutions; the environment, land, oil and other resources; health and disease; economy: growth, aid, taxation, debt and capital flight; and both Africa's international relations and country case studies.

Managing Editor, Stephanie Kitchen

Series editors

Adam Branch
Alex de Waal
Alcinda Honwana
Ebenezer Obadare
Carlos Oya
Nicholas Westcott

LESLIE BANK
NELLY SHARPLEY

Covid and Custom in Rural South Africa

Culture, Healthcare and the State

HURST & COMPANY, LONDON

IAI   International African Institute

Published in collaboration with the International African Institute.
First published in the United Kingdom in 2022 by
C. Hurst & Co. (Publishers) Ltd.,
New Wing, Somerset House, Strand, London WC2R 1LA
Copyright © Leslie Bank and Nelly Sharpley, 2022
All rights reserved.
Printed in the United Kingdom by Bell and Bain Ltd, Glasgow

The right of Leslie Bank and Nelly Sharpley to be identified as the
authors of this publication is asserted by them in accordance with the
Copyright, Designs and Patents Act, 1988.

A Cataloguing-in-Publication data record for this book
is available from the British Library.

ISBN: 9781787385733

This book is printed using paper from registered sustainable
and managed sources.

www.hurstpublishers.com

We are now in a war. We are in a war zone and our rights will inadvertently be affected and restricted for our own survival. ... The whole country is a hotspot on its own, including a number of areas where we thought the rate of infection would not be as big as in other areas.

South African President Cyril Ramaphosa, 16 July 2020

It is imperative South African elites wean themselves off the liberal notion of doing something "for the people" and embrace a people-centred model. ... Sustainable development is meaningful only if we do something "with the people". ... Development is only meaningful if it allows for the empowerment of communities to promote a spirit of self-reliance amongst the marginalised.

Zakes Mda, novelist, 1993[1]

CONTENTS

LIST OF MAPS, DIAGRAMS AND FIGURES

Maps

Diagrams

Figures

LIST OF MAPS, DIAGRAMS AND FIGURES

Map 1: Map of South Africa

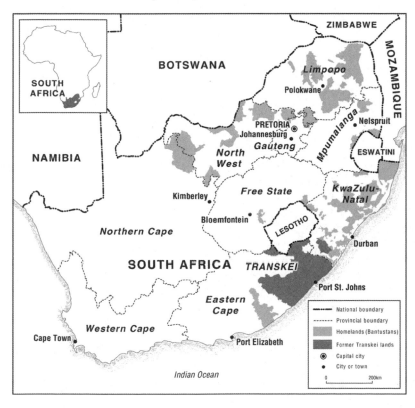

PREFACE AND ACKNOWLEDGEMENTS

This book grew out of a study that was initially imagined as a rapid rural appraisal project, commissioned by a government development agency in the Eastern Cape province of South Africa in April 2020. Its aim was to consider the impacts of lockdown restrictions on funerals and customary practices in rural communities in the former Transkei homeland of the province. The Eastern Cape Socio Economic Consultative Council (ECSECC) employed us to lead the project. We issued our initial report a month later, at the end of May, but due to the enthusiasm of the researchers, the complexity of the issues under investigation, and the difficulties in securing an ethical approval, the actual research continued for several months, allowing for a much deeper engagement with the topic and the rural communities than had initially been imagined.

Ten rural communities in the OR Tambo and the Chris Hani district municipalities were selected for the study, on the basis that these two districts were the leading hotspots for Covid-19 infections in rural South Africa at the time. Three locations were selected from Chris Hani and seven from OR Tambo, with the project covering several local municipalities: Intsika Yethu, Engcobo, Umhlontlo, Nyandeni, King Sabata Dalindyebo, Umzimvubu, Bizana and Ingquza. After the first wave of infections subsided in South Africa in July 2020, we wrote up a report and a policy brief, although the primary data collected for the project was quite substantial. In December 2020, as the second wave of infections swept through South Africa, we reassembled the research team with top-up funding from the

Human Sciences Research Council (HSRC), which kindly agreed to extend the project. The research for the second phase lasted until the end of January 2021, when the infection rate again came down. The second round of fieldwork was based in the same communities and we were able to follow up with families, village stakeholders and communities from the first phase. This gave the work depth and a longitudinal dimension, enabling us to track responses and experiences in the same places over time, something lacking from other research projects undertaken at this time.

Due to the threat of infection and lockdown restrictions, the data was collected using social networking, cellphones and observation at the village level. Researchers kept diaries of daily and weekly changes, which were compiled into situational analysis reports, and tracked every funeral held in these villages over several months. It was only much later, when ethical clearance for face-to-face interviews was acquired, that direct stakeholder interviews were possible. The great virtue of the delay in ethical approval was that it allowed us to coach the fieldworkers in observation and engaged-research techniques based on social networking and deploying cellphone technology. The research tools were designed to allow individuals and communities to express themselves in their own words, and in their own cultural idiom, on issues of concern. In a situation in which precious little reliable information was filtering down to the community level, the researchers themselves also offered a valuable source of information and a reference point for members of their communities. One of the unintended benefits of the project was that it enabled local people to access reliable information from the researchers about Covid-19, including about the nature of the virus and how it was transmitted. In this context, it is important to note that the researchers were selected because they were community insiders.

At a time when many Covid-19 research projects with a human sciences focus were based on telephone surveys, which tended to be conducted remotely, the project put people first and generated an on-the-ground perspective. It collected information in the language and categories of local people, using their social and cultural points of reference. Public interest in the research was considerable. The enforcement of new regulations on funerals, and the consequent infringement of cultural rights and the shutting down of customary practices, had become major talking points both in the national discourse and in local villages. Accordingly, the researchers allowed people to talk, and listened, often as third-party participants, to discussions which in many cases they had not initiated. The methodology was subtle, conversational and engaged.

Over the year, the status of traditional funerals and issues around the management of Covid-19 bodies after death became a national focus of interest. In this regard, the project and its findings also quickly attracted widespread attention. All the major national television and radio stations were keen to host us on news and talk shows. Between August 2020 and November 2020, the results of the research were shared on prime-time television and radio, including on SABC and eNews Channel Africa (ENCA), as well as on various community and local radio stations.

In addition to radio and television coverage at a national level, numerous op-eds were also published in influential print media outlets, such as the *Mail & Guardian* and the *Daily Maverick*, as well as on *African Arguments*, the insight platform of the International African Institute, based at SOAS University of London. The visibility achieved through this platform resulted in an offer to prepare a monograph for the African Arguments book series. The print media contributions were both descriptive and analytical, championing the value of "people's science" (see Introduction) and the need for the protection of cultural rights and human dignity, while at the same time sharing critical ethnographic and policy insights from the project. The strong policy focus has also been pursued in several sessions with government civil servants and policy makers, including the Eastern Cape House of Traditional Leaders and officials from the provincial Department of Health. A synopsis of the main policy conclusions is contained in an HSRC policy brief for public and government consumption. Three other short pieces were carried in the HSRC Review in 2020, one on the value of a people's science perspective; another on cultural dignity and Covid-19 funerals in rural villages; and a third on the failure of clinics and healthcare in rural communities during the crisis. The first draft of this book was produced at the end of April 2021, with a focus on the first year of the Covid experience in rural areas in South Africa.

The project has had a significant impact in the policy sphere. The integrity and quality of the research findings have lent weight to the need for a new, collaborative "people's science" approach to the management of the socio-cultural aspects of public health crises, such as that produced by the pandemic. A particular issue raised in the media and in our research was how new regulations introduced by the government on funerals and the handling of Covid-19 bodies had created widespread trauma and undermined the dignity and authenticity of Xhosa funeral rites. As a result, the provincial and national governments and the Ministerial Advisory Committee (MAC) on Covid-19 were urged to review the regulations pertaining to the viewing, protection and burial of bodies. In this context, it is a noteworthy achievement that the national government and MAC revised their advice on the handling of Covid-19 bodies in January 2021 in line with the recommendations produced by this research. The research has also been at the forefront of a campaign urging the government to show greater respect for the views of rural communities and display sensitivity to the cultural rights of marginalised communities when forging policy.

In terms of the acknowledgements, it is necessary to start by thanking Siv Hesjedal from ECSECC who responded to our request to source funding from the Eastern Cape government for a project investigating the response of rural communities to the lockdown restrictions on funerals and customary practices. She played a critical role in promoting the research and finding a wide audience for the results, including with traditional leaders and health professionals in the province. The communications expert, writer and policy specialist, Mark Paterson, was part of the core team during the ECSECC phase of the project and did a great deal of work compressing research notes and assisting us with writing and formulating the policy recommendations for government. He was the first to notice the disjuncture between the World Health Organization (WHO) recommendation for the treatment of Covid bodies and the approach adopted by the MAC. He also contributed to chapter five, "Gatekeepers". Aneza Madini, an HSRC researcher with excellent connection in the Engcobo area, also helped a great deal in tracking down cases of families who were exhuming bodies buried under Covid conditions and

PREFACE AND ACKNOWLEDGEMENTS

reburying them after lockdowns ended. The HSRC should also be acknowledged for recognising the value of the research undertaken in the first wave of the pandemic (March to July 2020) and agreeing to fund further research during the second wave.

Our greatest debt on this project is, however, to the fieldworkers from Walter Sisulu University, many of whom were senior students and staff in the Humanities, Social Sciences and Law faculty. The book would not have been possible without their accounts from behind lockdown lines, which documented the day-to-day events in rural locations and at funerals that family and friends attended. The team included Vuyiswa Taleni from Anthropology who did fieldwork in Lusikisiki; Mandlakazi Tshunungwa from Criminology in Intsika Yethu; Puleng Morori from Population Studies in King Sabata Dalinyebo; Buleka Shumane from Sociology in Mhlontlo; Athi Phiwane from Sociology in Mzimvubu; Zipho Xego from Sociology in Nyandeni; Siyasanga Fayini from Political Studies in Libode; Balindi Mayosi from Anthropology in Bashe; Phelisa Ellen Nombila from Criminolgy in Engcobo; and Singa Siyasanga from Environmental Sciences in Bizana. Finally, we thank our families for their support, patience and understanding in helping us get this book to press.

Finally, the production of this book would have not been possible without an invitation from the African Arguments series to transform our blogs on the Covid crisis in rural South Africa into a book. We thank them for that opportunity. We would also like to acknowledge the valuable and helpful comments of the two academic reviewers on the first draft. The book would still not have made it to print without the dedication, constant encouragement, and patient attention to detail of Stephanie Kitchen, our manging editor at the IAI at SOAS, and Alice Clarke and her team at Hurst for their steady support and professionalism throughout.

Leslie Bank and Nelly Sharpley
22 November 2021

INTRODUCTION

COVID AND CUSTOM

Most black people live undignified lives and only see dignity in death. Our freedom is in the afterlife and that is why we invest so much money in planning for our funerals. Covid-19 has taken this last shed of decency from us. It has stolen our rites of passage into heaven, we can't gather in the same way, or practise our traditions to properly send off our own and pay our last respects (except, of course, if you are some important government official, where the same rules do not seem to apply).

My mom was bundled up like trash, bound in plastic—she wasn't allowed (back) into her own yard (to say goodbye). We couldn't wash her or dress her to the nines for the last time, couldn't watch her body over in a night-time vigil or give her a final touch goodbye.

Paballo Chauke, "Thief in the Night: Covid took my Mom",
© *Mail & Guardian*, 19 January 2021

During funeral gatherings, Covid virus is [seen to be] caused by our customs, because the state is at war with us and our customs. We were chased by the police, together with the people who are supposed to govern us, and we had to run in confusion … the way these regulations are expressed and the law enforcement that accompanies them against funerals and customs is as if this was all caused by us.

Rural resident from the rural Eastern Cape, May 2020[1]

Introduction

On the last weekend of October 2021, a few days before the South African local government elections, a social media post went viral. It was a video of a family carting a coffin on an oxen-drawn sleigh along a dirt road in a remote district of the rural Eastern Cape. The coffin contained the body of a well-respected community leader, Mfomfomfo Mqala, who had died of natural causes at the age of 75 years and was being led to his final resting place at his village home-stead. The post was meant to highlight the ruling African National Congress (ANC) party's poor track record on service delivery and infrastructure development in rural areas during its 27 years in power. Viewers of the post noted how rural areas of the Eastern Cape always seemed to fall behind when other parts of the country moved forward. They wondered what icons of the ANC struggle from the region—like Nelson Mandela, Oliver Tambo, Govan Mbeki and Chris Hani—would have thought of the appalling state of rural infra-structure, the lack of jobs there and the routine hardship experienced by people in the former Transkei homeland in the Eastern Cape. The October social media post followed similar stories in the local media on the poor state of the roads and the difficulties families were expe-riencing at a time of many Covid deaths in the rural areas. The image of a coffin on a cart struggling along a rural road seemed like an appropriate depiction of the everyday struggles in rural areas, sym-bolising the devastating impact of the Coronavirus. Indeed, between March 2020 and March 2021, the Eastern Cape province recorded a Covid death rate of over 200 per 100,000, which was above the national average for the country and higher than the US, Italy or Brazil. The image of the coffin and the cart struck a chord because it was a story of death, disrespect and struggle at a particular time, and not just about the failure of municipal service delivery in rural areas. The post was powerful because of the way it revealed how rural people had been forgotten, disrespected and left out, especially dur-ing the Covid pandemic when tens of thousands died in the region. The video was shared repeatedly because of its striking incorporation of many aspects of rural distress and marginalisation.

On 5 November 2021, when the South African election results were officially reported on national television, it was clear that popu-lar trust and support for the ruling party had been severely dented since 2016. Voter turnout had dropped from half to around a third of the eligible voters and the support for the ruling liberation party fell by 10% across the country, with big losses registered in both urban and rural areas. The drop off in support in rural areas was hugely significant compared to previous elections, where there were very high levels of support for the ruling party in these areas. For residents in the homeland areas, the ANC was a liberation movement and the party of freedom from the clutches of apartheid: the system that entrapped them at home, and prevented them from taking jobs in urban areas without a pre-approved labour contract in an exploitative migrant labour system. In the 1990s, the ANC dismantled the system of enforced migrant labour, halted forced removals and reversed other aspects of the apartheid system. Rural people could move around freely throughout South Africa and were also paid social welfare grants and pensions, which had never been previously available in rural areas. They were also allowed to live on communal land in the rural setting without paying for services. By the 2010s, over two-thirds of rural households in the former homelands received billions of dollars in welfare support through social grants which were either transferred directly into bank accounts or collected at local service centres. Although rural voters complained of the lack of jobs and the poor state of infrastructure, the ANC was always eager to remind them of the welfare support that the state provided them with, and the importance of those resources to their survival and well-being in the countryside. In the 2016 local government elections, the ANC under the leadership of Jacob Zuma lost ground to other parties in the urban areas, but held the rural heartlands, where its support stood firm and even increased. By 2021, however, this was not the case; support had ebbed away considerably in these former strongholds. The low voter turnout and diminished government support was due to municipal service delivery failures and infrastructure deficits, but it was also fundamentally about the way the government had handled the Coronavirus crisis over the past 20 months.

The research for this book was undertaken in the former Transkei homelands of the rural Eastern Cape, where people used the phrase *ukuvala isango* ("closing the gate") to describe their experience of the government's handling of the Coronavirus crisis. This phrase was used across the region to refer not only to their sense of being materially left behind and excluded when others were able to move forward, but also in the sense of being confined to a place of spiritual insecurity, confusion and darkness by the actions the government in rural areas. *Ukuvala isango* carried multiple meanings. At one level, it literally referred to the closure of the garden gate during lockdown as families were restricted to their rural homesteads. However, it was also often used to reference the widespread closure of rural clinics and hospitals between April and July 2020, due to a lack of personal protective equipment and nurses and doctors refusing to work in unhygienic conditions. Others referred to the closure of many government departments as part of the general process of shutting down, including home affairs which usually issued death certificates. But *ukuvala isango* was also used to refer to the lack of communication about Covid in the rural areas, especially in the vernacular, or community campaigns to bring awareness about the virus to the people. The phase was also often invoked to describe the way in which the rules and regulations associated with the pandemic frightened them, and "closed the gate" on cultural practices and family lifecycle rites of passage due to the bans on customary practices such as funerals and other social occasions. Many families could not understand why the bodies—and even the coffins—of their loved ones were now sealed in plastic bags with stickers on them that could not be opened. They were also confused about why funeral parlour staff no longer brought the body of the deceased to their home before the funeral, but instead unceremoniously dumped it in the ground, "like trash", on the day of the funeral, while spraying the place with disinfectant and wandering around in white hazmat suits. Many wondered why they were being targeted in this way and told that their culture practices caused Covid, when they knew that the disease was brought into their areas from the outside. The original article picked up on social media read:

> Roads in one Eastern Cape village are so bad that a funeral parlour has to hire a donkey cart to take a coffin to the graveyard. In some instances, locals even use ladders as stretchers to carry departed relatives to their graves. The coffins are simply too heavy to do otherwise. The Covid-19 pandemic and its strict protocols mean burials have to take place quickly, but for years residents of Nyumaga village in Centane have been complaining about the state of their roads. That they have to use such drastic measures to lay their loved ones to rest is a disgrace, they told *Dispatch Live* on Tuesday.[2]

INTRODUCTION

The primary aim of this book is to reveal the meaning and experience of closing the gate (*ukuvala isango*) at both a material and spiritual level in rural communities, focusing on the former Transkei homeland of the Eastern Cape during the first and second waves of the Coronavirus pandemic. The research on which the book is based stems from ethnographic data collected from 10 locations within this region during the national lockdown of the first wave between April and July 2020. A second phase of research followed in the same areas during the second wave from December 2020 to January 2021, when the so-called South African variant of the virus swept through the country and spread to many parts of the world. The book thus tells the story of how marginalised communities on the rural periphery of South Africa experienced the first year of the Coronavirus crisis, paying particular attention to conditions in the rural Eastern Cape province. The book develops the argument that the South Africa government, encouraged by the private sector, opted for a first world bio-medical response to the Coronavirus crisis, in an attempt to to lead Africa in the world in its response. It could not support this approach scientifically, nor implement it bio-medically, outside of the middle-class suburbs in its main cities. The government decided to stand with the hegemonic bio-medical approach of the global North, which was supported by the suburban middle classes and political insiders in the ruling party; this decision occurred in a context where the state knew and understood that the model it adopted could only provide effective care for a small minority of the population. The political leadership knew that the majority of the population, especially the rural poor, had very limited access to the benefits of Western bio-medicine, or were compressed in urban township and shack areas where social distancing and middle-class hygiene standards were practically impossible. The argument of the book is that the state understood the disjuncture and contradictions in its policies and approach but nevertheless pushed through with the application of Western models to the enormous detriment of the poor in the country, who died in very large numbers and were generally excluded, marginalised and silenced. We suggest that the decision to follow the Northern middle-class bio-medical model rather than seek alliances and multiple perspectives, and promote more preventative approaches from below was taken with the recognition that, due to poverty and inequality in South Africa, the bio-medical system could only hope to effectively protect a small portion of its population.

Fear of the virus spreading rapidly across the entire population was also one of the reasons that the South Africa state adopted one of the toughest and longest lockdown periods in the world, which effectively lasted for five months, and severely limited the rights and freedoms of individuals to associate, travel or do business.[3] The prolonged lockdown was meant to buy time for the government to prepare its public health system for the first surge in infections in South Africa. By contrast to major Western democracies:

> Only 16 per cent of the South African population has access to medical aid, with most of its population relying on the public healthcare sector that is under resourced and poorly administered. In its 2016–2017 Annual Inspection Report, the Office of Health Standards reported that out of 851 public sector health establishments, 62 per cent of these were non-compliant with the norms and standards for healthcare quality. Areas of deficiencies identified included a lack of or poor leadership and management, knowledge, competencies, and support from senior staff.[4]

Thus, although the country presented itself to the international community as a modern state capable of maintaining a bio-medical regime of screening, testing, and isolating, it also realised it would be incapable of providing those services and resources to the whole population. This resulted in a situation where the state worked intensively on preparing its main metropolitan public hospitals and creating additional pop-up field hospitals with private sector support in the cities, while almost totally ignoring the upgrading of healthcare facilities in the rural areas, which generally had existing infrastructure and compliance problems. In this process, the state also rejected any alliance or engagement with popular movements and organisations, including traditional healers, and their associations as an alternative system of support in the fight against Covid infection. Instead, to "protect" the poor, the state turned instead to the police and the army to enforce the strict lockdown rules and regulations, resulting in hundreds of thousands of arrests or fines. Breaking the rules was deemed a criminal offence in terms of the Disaster Management Act of March 2020, which underpinned the hard lockdown instituted from midnight on the 26 March 2020 and maintained until August, when the first wave of infections started to fade. By June 2020, three months into lockdown, President Ramaphosa reported that the police had already made over 230,000 arrests for Covid related offences. The announcement was meant as a further warning to those who continued to disobey the law as Covid infections increased in South Africa. By February 2021, the Minister of Police in South Africa, Bheki Cele, said that over the previous year 411,309 people had been arrested for breaching lockdown regulations.[5] In the Eastern Cape province, almost 100,000 people were allegedly fined or prosecuted during the first year of Covid, many for breaching travel bans. However, large numbers of arrests were also made for breaches of the rules in relation to funeral regulations and the closure of initiation schools and customary practices.

In implementing its calibrated, top-down science model, the state adopted a strategy of "consultation" rather than engagement. The model was based on the idea that the knowledge that mattered for South Africa to minimise the impact of the Coronavirus would come from the scientific community, who would report to the President and his team so that the bio-medically driven approaches could be trickled down to the people with maximum effect. In the meantime, the government would continue to "consult" with leading stakeholders, like organised business, heads of hospitals and political parties, to assess opportunities for collaboration and resourcing in relation to the strategic direction adopted. These decisions were taken by the National Command Council, which implemented its decisions through a series of provincial and even district level command councils, created to ensure that all the decisions taken at the top could cascade down to all areas and communities. In the provinces, one of the critical local stakeholders and allies of the state were the houses of traditional leaders whose constituents lived in the communal areas of the former homelands. The state and its scientific advisors assumed that there would be low levels of compliance with the lockdown rules in these remote areas and felt that the traditional leaders and local police services had a key role to play in keeping rural communities in check. They also assumed that certain forms of social and cultural practices in these areas, based on the African philosophy of *ubuntu*

("I am because you are"), offered a special threat to containment. Indeed, the council figured that, if the social compression of life in poor urban areas presented a threat to government policy in the cities, the pursuit of customary practices in the countryside compounded this threat. In the minds of the political elites and their scientific advisors, customary funerals brought the dangers of the city to the countryside and were thus given special attention throughout the lockdown period.

The argument of this book is that, by virtue of their cultural and customary characteristics, certain rural areas, including those in the Eastern Cape, were elevated to a special level of danger. These areas were viewed through a particular lens which intensified the need for repression as the command council "calibrated" the risk of infection beyond the simple distinction between elites and the poor, or "the people" and the state.[6] We suggest that the experience of alienation, fear, and exclusion in certain rural places was thus qualitatively different from those in townships or shack areas, even though the level of poverty was similar. The purpose of this book is to bring these experiences out into the open, illuminating the way understandings of culture influenced state action in hidden places of suffering and repression in the time of the Covid pandemic. But the analysis provided is not restricted to a special kind of "expose" anthropology, which reveals the meanings and experience of this exclusion, suffering and alienation in faraway places; the book also aims to show how the customary practice and funerals specifically targeted by the state were themselves interwoven in the coping and livelihood strategies of the poor after apartheid. In this way, the book is ultimately able to offer a novel perspective on the cultural economy of poverty and inequality in South Africa today. Furthermore, the book is unique and original in that the fieldwork that informs the analysis was undertaken during lockdown, at a time where it was extremely difficult to conduct qualitative research in rural areas.

States of exception

In his 2021 book, *New Pandemics, Old Politics: Two Hundred Years of War on Disease and Its Alternatives*, Alex De Waal suggests that, while the dominant discourse around chronic diseases like diabetes centres on citizen responsibility, infectious diseases have generally allowed states to claim the initiative and mobilise a discourse of war in the name of protecting citizens from pathogens. This approach empowers states and potentially diminishes the possibilities for democratic public health, invoking a special kind of "bio-politics". The Italian philosopher Giorgio Agamben argued that, when the Covid-19 virus raged through Italy in March 2020 and the Italian state enforced extreme lockdown measures on the population, state officials deliberately created a "state of exception" where citizens' rights and freedoms were unnecessarily compromised.[7] He suggested that the authoritarian measures taken to confront the pandemic undermined democracy and could lead to fascism. He wrote of the "intimate solidarity between democracy and totalitarianism" and claimed the scale could easily tip in the wrong direction. Others disagreed, saying that such measures were necessary and only short-term.[8] In his new book, De Waal shows that the state authoritarianism that has historically come with new pandemics is the same "old politics" which lingers long after the pandemic subsides.[9] But others have argued that Covid is no ordinary flu and that Agamben's call for freedom is unreasonable and ill-conceived.[10]

Contemporary life, in the concept of biopolitics proposed by Agamben, has become a bare life. Life thus conceived is reduced to what is produced and managed by law. The individuals in the Nazi concentration camps, where the most reprehensible cruelty took place under state power and order, were stripped of all rights and political-legal status; their life was treated, by the agents of power, as matter without human form, creating a 'naked life' where they were simply data, figures, biological units that were always disposable. Agamben opposed this condition to greater value that existed for other lives, that were preserved and extended by the suffering and ultimate extermination of those confined to naked life. Under the rule exercised by a system of power, Agamben argues that human life is pauperised in general but also annihilated. Among the concentration camp subjects, Agamben focuses on two different figures, those that are resigned to dying, engulfed in humiliation, fear, and horror, on the one hand, and the condition of the *homo sacer*, persons of low status and general invisibility, first defined under Roman law, who were banned and could be killed but not sacrificed. They were trapped in what he called a bare life, between the elites with escalating state power and privilege and those who lived the naked life.[11]

This triadic conceptualisation of bio-power and vulnerability in the context of Western culture and state formation clearly has wider applicability in the global context of inequality; it is also applicable in the time of Covid, where hegemonic Northern models have been widely adopted in the global South. In South Africa, for example, the state opted for one of the toughest lockdown regimes in the world, which was extended for six months. On 5 March 2020, Minister of Health Zweli Mkhize confirmed the spread of the virus to South Africa. On 15 March, the President of South Africa, Cyril Ramaphosa, declared a national state of disaster, and announced measures such as immediate travel restrictions and the closure of schools from 18 March. On 17 March, the National Coronavirus Command Council was established, "to lead the nation's plan to contain the spread and mitigate the negative impact of the coronavirus". On 23 March, a national lockdown was announced, starting on 27 March 2020. From 1 June, the national restrictions were lowered to level 3. The restrictions were lowered to alert level 2 on 17 August 2020, bringing life back to a measure of normalcy. From 21 September 2020, restrictions were again lowered to alert level 1. The restrictions were, however, raised again in December 2020, when fatalities spiked as a result of a second wave of infection driven by the more infectious "South African variant".[12]

In this book, we argue that those living at the margins in the former South Africa homelands—in the past compared to concentration camp interns, especially under apartheid rule—were once again bought to the edge of naked life, as Chauke's opening quote suggests.[13] They were like trash to be cast aside. Indeed, this book hopes to illustrate how the application of a "greater" state of exception in these rural places meant that the humiliation, fear, horror, and undignified death associated with Covid was compounded by a combination of control, repression and exclusion that undermined the very possibility of social reproduction. It was, however, not just the rule of law and the force of the state that brought such dire conditions into existence, but also the systematic neglect of the promise of care and protection which the state extended in March 2020, with its declaration of a national State of Disaster. The book focuses on the experience of the first year of these conditions, which have lessened at the time of writing, but could always be ramped up again to deal with a renewed outbreak of the virus.

In his historical work, Alex De Waal shows that metaphors of war and fighting have centrally shaped the way in which modern states have responded to pandemics over the past 200 years. His intriguing history of pandemics since cholera in the mid-19th century suggests that war and disease are, in fact, closely intertwined, although this is seldom recognised in the heroic nationalist histories that describe major conflicts.[14] For example, De Waal suggests that in the Crimean War and the First World War, more people in the trenches and on the frontlines died as disease fodder than as cannon fodder. Indeed, military leaders had such a good understanding of the power of disease in war that, in previous centuries, they were even known to project infected bodies across enemy lines as a deliberate strategy of war.[15] The role of disease in histories of conflict has been hugely under-played and has only recently been revealed by health historians and medical anthropologists. De Waal argues that the metaphor of "fighting" a disease, apt for the body's immune response to a pathogen, has also been adopted by modern states to suspend the rights, freedoms, and liberties of citizens in the name of the collective effort to contain and restrict infection.[16] When mobilising for war, states resort to authoritarian measures as "political leaders inveigh against 'infestation' by invaders or infiltrators that are akin to pathogens and, in times of health crisis, they like to 'declare war' on a microbial 'invisible enemy'." De Waal claims that, while governments often insist that the medical crisis is unique and specific, the historical evidence suggests that once states "declare war", they lay claim to special powers and resources to manage the crisis. These interventions tend to make greatly expanded state power and authoritarianism a legacy of pandemics.[17]

The response of the modern state to plagues or pandemics has also favoured a discourse of *inclusion* by presenting the threat as affecting all citizens. The state insists that the threat posed by pathogens is not limited to one segment of the population, a single social class or race group, but is a threat against the nation itself. As such, the state must mobilise to protect all citizens irrespective of their social and economic standing or where they are located. The need to include all citizens and marginal groups is how states then justify the need for special allocations of public funds during pandemics. In his reflections on the emergence of "abnormality" in modern Western society, the French philosopher Michel Foucault noted that, with modernity, European states moved away from the desire to separate the sick from the healthy, as expressed in the model of the leper colony, and embraced techniques of power that sought to observe, analyse and control human beings in order to individualise and normalise them.[18] This shift was entrenched in new responses to plagues, leading Foucault to argue that the modern subject was manufactured in part by state management of disease and biopolitics.[19] Under Covid, many states have attempted to individualise citizen responses and normalise self-discipline, while at the same time assuming that not all citizens are equally capable or equipped to behave "responsibly". Minority groups, migrants and traditional communities or "first nations" have been targeted for "special treatment" to bring them in line with what is assumed to be the more modernised response of urban populations, especially the middle classes. In terms of the leper colony metaphor, they are still seen to exist outside of modernity and in need of special treatment to normalise their behaviour and moderate their response.

This is exactly what happened as the Covid-19 outbreak in China became a global pandemic in 2020. A hegemonic discourse of war on disease became globally pervasive as politicians called for states to have "war-time emergency powers"—special rights to manage and control populations and to survey the behaviour of citizens—and access to public funds to dispense special packages that would stimulate growth, address infection and support vulnerable groups. In the United States, President Donald Trump was quick to call himself a "war-time president", following the statement by the French President Emmanuel Macron that France would declare a war on the virus. In Hungary, the populist leader Viktor Orbán passed laws allowing him to rule by decree indefinitely and blamed the pandemic on immigrants and refugees.[20] In China, the lockdown was enforced by a combination of hi-tech, smart-city surveillance and old-fashioned

Communist party neighbourhood mobilisation, under which city grids could be broken down for effective surveillance. A similarly hi-tech approach, developed to combat terror attacks, was adopted in Israel, while Italy, which lacked surveillance technologies, relied on enhanced police powers. However, it is also striking to note the differences between the state's expectations of citizens in protectionist, liberal-welfarist regimes and in populist ones.

In Trump's America, where the success of the economy was placed ahead of the health of the nation, citizens were encouraged not to wear masks and to continue their normal lives so as not to disrupt the economy. Thus, while Trump declared war on the pandemic, his government did not seek to promote or enforce tight controls on citizens, which led to extensive criticism of his response among the urban middle classes. In Britain, by contrast, the Conservative Party under Boris Johnson ultimately adopted a strongly welfarist, health-centred approach with tight regulations on citizens and extensive social support for poor and vulnerable groups. In Sweden, the state acknowledged the severity of the pandemic but adopted a minimalist approach, allowing citizens to manage themselves as modern, responsible, self-regulating subjects. Overall, the health-centred, welfarist approach in which the state enforced tough lockdown restrictions on citizens for extended periods in 2020 emerged as the dominant model in Europe and Latin America, although countries like Brazil and the US opted for an approach which prioritised the economy instead of the pandemic.

In South Africa, the pandemic arrived at a time when corruption and political factionalism within the ANC was undermining the legitimacy of the ruling party and the state. The Covid-19 crisis thus provided an opportunity for the ruling faction within the party, under President Cyril Ramaphosa, to seize the initiative and reassert their connection to the global North by declaring their own war on the pathogen and designing a rational, health-centred, population-control response from the state. The Disaster Management Act of March 2020 was deployed to declare a state of disaster and a Ministerial Advisory Committee (MAC) of high-level medical experts and scientists was appointed to advise the President on the changing nature of the threat and the measures needed to contain it. In the absence of hi-tech surveillance or reliable community-level structures to assist the state with monitoring and surveillance, the response was centralised in the Office of the Presidency and framed as a universal set of measures for all citizens, rich and poor, urban and rural. A military-style National Coronavirus Command Council was also established, and the provinces were required to submit regular updates the Minister of Health, Zweli Mkhize, the MAC and Ramaphosa. In his speeches, the President stressed that the success of the tough lockdown regime would rest on citizen compliance, which made it necessary for the police and army to assist with implementation across the nation.

By choosing to upgrade the Disaster Management Act rather than declaring a national state of emergency, the President and his team of advisers ensured that they had access to institutional mechanisms for the creation of command centres in all provinces and districts. This system potentially created a mechanism for the dissemination of information up and down the hierarchy from the district level to the presidency. This mechanism for inter-governmental relations was primarily intended to disseminate the rules and instructions of the President, the Minister of Health and their team of advisors to the provinces and districts. The first meeting between the provincial councils and the President only occurred in May, two months after lockdown was announced, indicating that the provincial and district councils served primarily as implementation agencies. But there was one area where the President and his team needed cooperation from the provincial councils right at the outset, and this was in controlling rural funerals and customary practices, which were assumed to present a major threat to the containment of the virus. The provincial government of the Eastern Cape, with the support of the regional house of traditional leaders, placed a blanket ban on the performance of customary practices from March 2020. In the eyes of the National Command Council, the Eastern Cape was a national centre for customary practices, including large traditional funerals and male initiation schools, that could serve as "super spreaders" of the virus. During the first year of Covid, it was not President Ramphosa but Dr Nkosazana Dlamini-Zuma—Minister of Cooperative Governance and Traditional Affairs—who made the main announcements concerning changes in regulations, especially in relation to customary practices, funerals and social distancing. However, Ramaphosa continuously urged people to stay away from customary events, saying that "funerals have become a death trap for many of our people. For now, it is best and safer to stay at home".[21]

In Giorgio Agamben's terms then, the South Africa state enforced a "state of exception" like that declared in Italy and western Europe by suspending individual rights so that the state could better fight the war on Covid.[22] However, unlike in Italy and other countries in the global North, the South African state was quick to announce that it was necessary not only to suspend individual rights, but also to cancel all customary practices, especially those associated with rural funerals. In this way, the South African state created a special category of exception, applicable to certain socio-cultural categories and groups that lived in cultural enclaves in the former homeland or Bantustans. In these places, it was assumed that the danger of contagion lay not only in the potential for deviant individual behaviour, but in custom and culture as well. The late doctor and activist Paul Farmer has written extensively on the pathologies of power in contexts where Western medicine, colonialism and neo-liberal economics intersect, allowing experts to repackage unacceptable inequalities in service delivery and care as the product of cultural difference—rather than structural violence—in post-colonial settings.[23] French historian and anthropologist Florence Bernault has also written that for Africa: "Covid-19 has [again] brought out [the image of] an allegedly under-medicalised, pre-modern Africa", which is seen as poverty-stricken, inherently under-developed and medically impotent in the face of disease.[24] Indeed, when the Covid-19 crisis in Asia became a global pandemic, Melinda Gates of the Bill & Melinda Gates Foundation said that she could not sleep at night because she feared the devastation that the Coronavirus might cause across the African continent, which "lacked the capacity to protect itself" from the deadly surge of the virus which was already gripping much of the rest of the world.

The political scientist, Steven Friedman, has also depicted the Covid response in South Africa as colonialist, arguing that the ruling class has been colonised by a high modernist scientific approach that assumes that clever people are best equipped to act on behalf of those with less knowledge and understanding.[25] He suggests that once this type of civilising mission was adopted with the support of business and the suburban middle classes, the state cast its gaze downwards on the townships and poor people who were assumed to be ignorant, irresponsible and lacking in the essential self-discipline and self-regulation needed to respond in a preventative manner to the pandemic.[26] For this reason, he suggests, the focus on state intervention in poorer areas focused on control and repression rather than care or protection. He stresses that while there was one virus there were essential two countries that were being served with different regimes.[27] In the suburbs and upper-class areas citizens were assumed to have some rights and were consulted and engaged with on key issues of policy and protection, while in the poorer parts of the country, especially the townships, shack lands and rural areas, the focus was almost exclusively on control. In Agamben's terms some citizens were able to retain more rights than others. Friedman argues that the way the state was able to construct the poor as irresponsible and essentially "uncivilised" made it much easier for them to suspend rights in these areas than in others without good reason or concern for recourse. Friedman suggest that since the state was only prepared to consult with lobbies—like business, labour, and political parties—those who did not have access to lobby groups to represent their interests were essentially forgotten.

There is much wisdom and insight in Friedman's analysis, but it does not give sufficient attention to the way politicians and experts differentiated amongst the poor, when calibrating the potential threat and danger to the nation that different categories of poor people posed. This is precisely where older notion of "civilised" insiders and "tribal" outsiders were reconstructed as filters for the perception of danger and risk, as Florence Bernault suggests in her review of Covid and colonial science.[28] In the early 2010s, such ideas had gained traction with the multiple outbreaks of Ebola, also a coronavirus, in West and Central Africa. Although the virus was regionally contained and proved much less widespread than other similar virus outbreaks in Asia, such as SARS, the World Health Organization (WHO) panicked and assumed that the Ebola virus would run riot across the continent and escape into western Europe with devastating effects. The global response to the threat posed by Ebola was urgent and immediate, and involved the creation of multiple field hospitals across the region which deployed the most advanced bio-technical interventions that were available.

By 2015, however, local-level preventative interventions forged by communities in coordination with international doctors, as well as the introduction of effective home-care regimes, had contained the virus. The fear subsided, although the Northern discourse of African ignorance, cultural otherness and lack of modernity did not.[29] With these narratives close at hand, the arrival of the so-called South African and Brazilian variants of Covid-19 started to spread infection in the global North at the end of 2020. In Britain and elsewhere in the global North, there was a sudden shift in the tone of international media coverage and political discourse. Well-worn colonial stereo-types came to the fore: images of Africa (and subsequently India given the "Indian" or Delta variant) as a perpetual threat to the public health and hygiene of modern industrial and civilised nations. Thinly veiled racism in the media exaggerated the danger posed by the African variant, invoking the old colonial discourse of death and disease ema-nating from the "dark continent". A similar discourse emerged in the global North around the "Brazil variant", which is often discussed in tandem with its South African cousin. In South Africa, the former homelands acquired the image of the "colonial other" with the poten-tial to drive infections into the stratosphere through the cultural agency of rural people who were unable to modernise their behav-iours in response to the pandemic. This created an even further state of exception, which required specialised state intervention.

Public health and people's science

In *New Pandemics, Old Politics* Alex De Waal argues that the hegemonic discourse of war on pathogens, which builds and sustains authoritarian states, never succeeds in fully overcoming the threat of infectious disease, even when effective vaccinations are developed to stop viruses from spreading.[30] The pathogens survive and continue to spread, while the actual conditions that created the disease in the first place are never addressed. De Waal insists that longer term, sustain-able solutions to the recurring crisis of infectious disease require more democratic and inclusive systems of public health and knowledge-sharing about the causes and containment of disease. This cannot simply be an issue of state-enforced interventions to minimise biological transmission, maximise individual self-regulation and pursue a curative solution in the form of a vaccine. Such a limited approach entrenches the power of the state and strips public health of its social context because diseases are transmitted, understood, and experienced within a wider ecology of social relationships, practices, and beliefs. Understanding and addressing this ecology is critical to longer-term strategies for prevention and sustainable environmental management. De Waal argues that the efficacy of sustainable, longer-term interventions is limited by the failure of states to generate what he terms "people's science" (borrowing from Paul Richards, see below)—where consensus is reached through the open exchange of ideas as well as scientific and local knowledge. Without engagement and the co-production of new knowledge and joint strategies, people inevitably go back to the same destructive behaviours that produce pandemics in the first place, which also limits the efficacy of vaccines in their capacity to remove the threat of disease.[31]

Paul Richards has argued that the power of "people's science" in addressing disease in Africa is hugely under-estimated because Western medical experts fail to recognise the capacity of local people to adjust their behaviour in relation to new evidence; they also tend to view local cultural beliefs and social practices as dangerous to disease transmission rather than an opportunity through which more effective and democratic preventative practices can be crafted.[32] In the case of Ebola, Richards found that once local communities in West Africa had engaged openly with medical experts and government officials, they realised that the diseased Ebola bodies were highly infectious and that transmission spread through touching and cleaning bodies. They were then quite prepared to change their home-care regimes and funeral practices to minimise the risk of infection and transmission. This allowed homes and villages to be transformed into safer spaces and made a massive contribution to the containment of Ebola in West Africa, where formal state health infrastructure, like hospitals and clinics, were and are in short supply. In short, by democratising the practice of prevention and disease control, and embedding it in a local ecology of social and cultural relationships which extended beyond the state, the hospital and the clinic, the capacity for control and prevention was improved and ultimately containment became possible. In the West African case, the approach emerged partly because of the weakness of states to enforce a local or national war on Ebola and their reliance on international bodies like the WHO to lead the "fight" by providing expertise and funds. Weak West African states, such as Sierra Leone, seemed to lack the resources and capacity to declare war on Ebola. However, it was precisely in this lacuna that people were able to work with foreign doctors and non-governmental organisations (NGOs) to share knowledge and create practical strategies, which were then later adopted by local government agencies.

The response to Covid-19 in South Africa has been quite different. The national government followed the Northern modernist, strong-state model by activating a "war on Covid". Local cultural practices were deemed dangerous, deviant and in need of being curtailed or suspended; they were replaced by the implementation of a universal code for individual behavioural adjustments based on bio-medical science. The President and health minister were led in their decision-making by teams of medical scientists and bio-medical experts, who were generally following global science and international best practices, rather than engaging with local social scientists, civic organisations, and cultural leaders in forging their behavioural prescriptions. By the end of April 2020, there were still no social scientists, cultural specialists, religious leaders, or community representatives on the MAC;[33] and yet a great deal of what the committee proposed in the opening months of the Covid crisis was the enforced suspension of cultural practices. In line with this approach, the government deemed funerals to be "super spreader" events which could only take place with restrictions on the numbers attending, the management of the ritual and the handling of the body. The rules stated that family or mourners should not engage with the bodies of the deceased, which should be wrapped in plastic to prevent infection among immediate family who might be inclined to touch or wash the corpse at home before placing the coffin in the earth. In the course of 2020, and especially as the rates of infection increased, the state and its scientific

19

committee remained adamant that the bodies of the deceased were the most dangerous elements at funerals and that they should be sealed to protect mourners.

This discourse of the body had a profound impact on the way in which funeral parlours operated and set out to protect their own workers, who handled dead bodies every day. To avoid unnecessary infection, it was decided by the state with funeral parlours that bodies should be wrapped in multiple layers of plastic when they left the mortuary and should only be delivered to the grave site on the day of the funeral and not before. In some provinces, such as the Eastern Cape, it was additionally decided that all bodies should be tested to determine whether they were Covid-19 deaths or not. At the same time families who hosted funerals were required to keep attendance registers and offer sanitising stations and appropriately spaced seating to allow the events to meet government standards. Funeral services were also to be no longer than two hours, during which time the body would arrive and be deposited at the grave site by the funeral parlour workers. Night vigils at which the family would engage with the deceased were strictly banned, as was the practice of the body lying at rest in a tent where the funeral service was held and where people paid their last respects.

Paul Richards' 2016 book, *Ebola: How People's Science Helped End an Epidemic*, provides a powerful reminder of the limits of epidemiology and bio-medical fixes, such as lockdowns, in the long-term control, management and elimination of diseases such as Covid-19.[34] Richards shows that, while the global North's bio-medical regime was developing vaccine trials and new nanotechnologies, and even imagining robotic nurses as potential strategies against Ebola, ordinary people in West Africa were paying careful attention to the technology of the infected body. They quickly came to learn how contagious and deadly the disease was, killing nine out of every ten people infected. They adjusted their regimes of behaviour in home-care, changing the ways they interacted with sick people, behaved at funerals and buried their dead. Richards shows how a "people's science" of behaviour and understanding emerged in a context-specific way. This was mediated through adjustments to local cultural practices and social values, to ultimately defeat a disease that Western medical science could not overcome.

INTRODUCTION

In his writing on people's science, Richards stresses that the preventative strategies that emerged at household and community levels in West Africa were not the product of rural people using indigenous knowledge and cultural beliefs *against* Western bio-medical and scientific knowledge, but were the result of a process of "co-production" based on all available evidence at the local level. People's science in this reading is conceived as an evidence-based system of adjustments in local social and cultural practices to accommodate the realities of a highly infectious and deadly disease, which was both novel and frightening. Richards challenges the dominant Eurocentric presumption that Africans in rural settings with limited formal education and exposure to Western scientific knowledge would respond to the crisis out of ignorance, or through a slavish adherence to local cultural beliefs. His position challenged the orthodox developmentalist stance that it was all about more hospitals, technical bio-medical equipment and highly trained doctors and medical scientists.[35] The perception of Africans as ignorant and culturally conservative, or unreceptive to change and entrapped in their traditional beliefs systems has a long history, making Richards' argument and observations novel and informative.

But the kinds of local cultures of prevention that emerged in certain parts of West Africa during Ebola were not generally replicated in rural South Africa once it became democratic, even though the government has promoted primary healthcare and community engagement at a policy level. The expectation of citizens has been that the state will and should intervene to provide a credible basic public health system which upholds their constitutional rights to decent healthcare services. The common understanding has been that the state will lead, and citizens should follow. There have been some significant achievements: the expanded infrastructure of clinics across rural areas and the roll-out of anti-retroviral drugs to fight the devastation wrought by HIV and AIDS. In relation to curative strategies, productive interactions with communities and different kinds of home-care systems have also been established, including those funded by USAID for the treatment and management of HIV and AIDS sufferers. However, the formal public health system has not sought to integrate traditional healing and the indigenous health and welfare

21

sector, which has remained outside its parameters; and, notwith-standing several ambitious policy pledges, the massification of public health in rural areas has been far less successful than many imagined it would be. More broadly, the types of interventions which have been implemented differ markedly from those envisaged by the idea of a people's science, which should be generated from the bottom by communities actively taking on board the evidence of bio-medicine and Western science to find locally appropriate solutions.

State services and infrastructure in rural South Africa are better than in many parts of West Africa. For example, there are clinics in almost every district and welfare grants are distributed by the state to about two-thirds of all rural households. In this context, most rural people believe that the state has the resources and will eventually deliver the required basic services to their communities. Thus, if they are dissatisfied their main approach is to exert pressure on the rele-vant officials or department to deliver what has been promised. In South Africa, there is still the expectation that the state will eventu-ally provide the service. It is therefore deemed not necessary, or even appropriate, for people to take matters into their own hands and co-produce knowledge or strategies that compete with or contradict the state's efforts in rural areas. Such blending is also not encouraged by the state, nor seen as something that the government would sup-port in local communities. Instead, when the official systems fail, people tend to rely more heavily on traditional healers and other service providers whom they often consult while also accessing ser-vices from the formal health system. The most common approach chooses from a range of different strategies at different times and in different circumstances, instead of actively trying to construct a people's science which adapts the prescriptions of the bio-medical approach to meet local health care needs.

AIDS denialism and the bio-medical fix

In the 1990s, the anthropologist Nancy Scheper-Hughes produced an unsettling ethnography of death, violence and hope in a shantytown in north-eastern Brazil. Her book, *Death Without Weeping: The Violence of Everyday Life in Brazil*, was centrally concerned with how shockingly high levels of infant mortality were hidden from public view by the ways in which women and families coped with this reality in the community.[36] Scheper-Hughes noted that young women in this place were refusing to name their children to protect themselves and their families from the pain of having to deal with the full, pervasive impact of death. She argued that by delaying the attribution of social and cultural identities to children, such as through naming, baptism and other rites, these mothers were better prepared to deal socially, financially and emotionally with the almost inevitable loss of one or more of their infants. The "people's science" of the Brazilian favela did not stop infant mortality because it was unstoppable within a political economy which left poor, vulnerable women without food and healthcare. In this context, women had no way of saving their children so they developed a practice of refusing to name their own children to help themselves cope with their likely deaths. Scheper-Hughes' ethnography tells a harrowing tale of the failure of "people's science" to make any significant impact in mitigating the structural constraints of shanty life in north-eastern Brazil.

The story of HIV and AIDS in South Africa bears some comparison with Scheper-Hughes's case study. The evidence from South Africa during the HIV and AIDS pandemic suggests that the country initially went down the road of official denialism and cultural concealment rather than confrontation. The internalisation of the bio-medical implications of HIV and AIDS was slow in South Africa, starting with the Thabo Mbeki regime's AIDS denialism, when the state questioned the core findings of the dominant Western bio-medical model. But even after the state acknowledged that HIV and AIDS was not just a disease of poverty and that it could not be cured by improved nutrition, there was still widespread popular denialism through folk theories of causality and connection. These varied from rumours and beliefs that traditional healers could "AIDS-proof" people through treatment, to ideas that condoms caused rather than prevented the spread of HIV and AIDS.[37]

One of the critical issues in the case of HIV and AIDS in southern Africa has always been the associated shame, and the reluctance of families to disclose the actual cause of death. Obituaries seldom mentioned AIDS and death notices were carefully worded to disguise any association with the dreaded disease. Those who were grievously ill were often removed from the cities and sent to die in the countryside. Deploying folk models around causation, which challenged the Western bio-medical model of personal or individual blame, people were simply not prepared to accept that their behaviour could make them vectors for the disease, instead attributing its spread to other factors. The net result was a kind of "death without weeping", or "invisible genocide", in which the extent of the disease's death toll was hidden or concealed from view, and even refuted. This did not make the impact of the deaths any less traumatic for the families, nor did it free them of the financial and social burden of caring for the sick and burying the dead, but it did help them deal with the question of shame and dishonour.

As a consequence, and despite the considerable impact of AIDS activism in South Africa, no effective "people's science" was developed to stop the spread of HIV in the country, even though the South African state eventually turned its back on denialism and adopted an extremely proactive, supportive set of policies and strategies.[38] In his recent book on the transition from AIDS denialism to the anti-retroviral drugs revolution in rural South Africa, Jonathan Stadler notes that the shift in policy had a profound effect on rural mortality rates in rural areas, which returned to pre-AIDS levels in many areas after the ARV drugs became universally available—even in remote areas, like Bushbuckridge in the former Lebowa homeland. Stadler argues that, while the stigma associated with having AIDS has remained and silence persists in relation to the disease, the miraculous effectiveness of anti-retroviral therapies (ART) has generated great optimism and hope. ART has saved lives and rehabilitated people and communities, as bio-medicine conquers the challenge of AIDS. The optimistic discourse is not confined, Stadler notes, to doctors, pharmaceutical companies and the Department of Health—which has played a vital role in ensuring that the ART is widely available—but is also embraced by ordinary people who speak of the new era, the ART epidemic. Bio-medical therapies have changed their lives, making those who were once downtrodden now able, optimistic and alive. Through bio-medical intervention, it is alleged that AIDS infection has changed from a terminal condition to a chronic illness. Stadler thus writes that the "biological effects of ART have rendered the disease undetectable", which therefore continues to generate discourses that deny the existence of AIDS and the suffering it has caused. In other words, it perpetuates the practices of silent death and suffering, what Scheper Hughes called "death without weeping".

Anthropologists like Jonathan Stadler, Isak Niehaus and Patricia Henderson have tried to break through the bio-medical story of success and the perceived ART revolution in South Africa. They aim to expose the continued presence and impact of HIV and AIDS on everyday lives in poor and marginalised communities in South Africa, underpinned by what Paul Farmer would call suffering and structural violence. These scholars also emphasis the extent to which individuals and rural communities operate in registers other than those of the pervasive individualised, curative bio-medical discourse; rural communities continue to use the idioms of witchcraft and other moral and cultural discourses to make meaning of their experiences. The fact that AIDS remains a "public secret" does not mean that it is insignificant in the minds and lives of those who suffer with it. While this is perhaps not the place to delve further into the hidden personal worlds and ongoing struggles with the AIDS pandemic in South Africa, it does seem clear that at a formal and political level the ART pill-driven revolution has been regarded as bio-medical triumph and fix for one of the most devastating diseases to have gripped southern Africa. However overstated and ideologically driven this may seem, it is a message that reshaped the AIDS industry and the official perception of the power of bio-medicine in South Africa. It also helps to explain why, when faced with the Covid crisis in 2020, the South African state and its public health system responded by turning so quickly to the Northern bio-medical establishment for guidance and direction. Hence, while there were practical reasons—such as the existence of relatively robust bio-medical and science systems in the metropolitan centres—one should not under-estimate the power of the ART revolution, the consolidation of the AIDS industry and its ideological influence when considering the South African state's choices when it came to Covid-19.

From the outset of the global Covid-19 pandemic, as noted above, governments around the world have generally failed to turn to their citizens for their views and advice, or included them proactively in strategies to combat the pandemic. In the global 2020–21 crisis, states have assumed that the social instincts of their citizens, particularly in the context of compressed urban lives, require close management and restriction to minimise transmission of the Coronavirus. But there has also been considerable debate about the reasons for differing transmission rates between countries with similar socio-economic profiles, polices and approaches. For example, why have thirty times more people died in Mexico than in Japan, even though both countries adopted similar polices and both have a population of around 100 million people? Why have the rates of infection been so much higher in Brazil and America than in other states? And why has South Africa had such high inflection rates relative to other countries on the African continent, when it has employed very strict policies of lockdown and government control?

In his 2009 book on AIDS in Africa, *Unimagined Community*, Thornton argues that one of the reasons that HIV and AIDS spread so rapidly in South Africa relative to other African countries was the relative openness (or "looseness") of sexual networks there.[39] In Uganda, by contrast, Thornton argued that ethnic and clan affiliation and social hierarchies restricted sexual networks, making targeting and treatment of the virus and disease easier. In his analysis, Thornton suggests the response to the pandemic was often based on a Eurocentric moralism, as we are now seeing with Covid. This moralism focused on individual behaviour, such as the need for monogamy and condom use, rather than a broader cultural understanding of kinship and social relatedness.[40] The apparent greater social cohesion or "tightness" of rural culture might thus have been viewed as an opportunity and resource, as it was in Sierra Leone during the Ebola pandemic, to build strong preventative strategies with local social and political legitimacy. In the view of the South African state, the existence of nodes of social cohesion in rural areas—what the President once called the culture of *ubuntu*—has generally been perceived as a threat to the containment of Covid. The assumed super spreader capacity of African culture, especially in rural areas, has encouraged the President and his team of scientific advisers to persistently and relentlessly highlight rural funerals and customary practices as the gravest threats to the national effort to flatten the inflection curve. In the words of one rural resident in the former Transkei, when the government speaks it is like "our culture and customs caused Covid, when we all know that it is disease that comes from somewhere outside South Africa".[41]

Migrant culture and homemaking

This book is concerned with custom and culture and its relationship to Covid-19 in the rural areas of South Africa. It considers the impacts of the pandemic and the responses to it in these areas, insofar as they are sites for homemaking and social reproduction which rely on customary practices and especially ritual activity to effect cohesion. Materialist writings on the rural periphery of South Africa have tended to see the hinterland of the infamous colonial and apartheid migrant labour system (and also former Bantustans) merely as African "labour reserves", created and maintained by white capital and the colonial/apartheid state. One school of thought argued that the homelands or Bantustans were initially beneficial for the development of a market economy in South Africa, but became increasingly dysfunctional to the country's capitalist development by inhibiting growth, especially during the apartheid period.[42] These scholars argued that if rural people in the "native reserves", or homelands, were given the choice, they would have moved to the cities in massive numbers after the Second World War, when South Africa experienced sustained secondary industrialisation.[43] In this view, the apartheid policies were uniquely punitive, racist and irrational, preventing migrants and peasant farmers from naturally urbanising and improving their lives. A counter argument to this view was produced by neo-Marxist scholars, who rose to prominence in South Africa in the 1970s and 1980s. They maintained that ever since the discovery of minerals in South Africa in 1870s, a system of racial capitalism had developed where the wealth of the white colonial ruling class depended on the exploitation of cheap labour from the reserves through a system of migrant labour. In this analysis, from the outset, the maintenance of male circular migration was functional rather than dysfunctional to the accumulation of capital by the white bourgeoisie;

and was thus maintained and reinvented to serve the dominant interests. Under this view, apartheid policies simply modernised and restructured older systems of labour management which underpinned the profits and power relations produced by racial capitalism.[44]

In the debates from this era, liberals shared the view of the Marxists that African men and women in rural areas had a strong desire to urbanise and establish themselves as a mature industrial working class with full civil and political rights and access to family wages in the towns and cities. But there were also some Africanists who resisted the easy comparisons between industrialising South Africa and developments in Europe. Archie Mafeje and Bernard Magubane, for instance, rejected the idea that upwardly mobile Africans simply aimed to mimic European lifestyles and identities by acquiring better jobs in town, becoming Christianised and participating more actively in consumer society. Mafeje argued that migratory Africans in rural areas were always more interested in acquiring and exchanging livestock, which underpinned their kinship system and social hierarchies, than in arable farming which the colonial government promoted so that migrant families could feed themselves outside the capitalist system. He rejected the idea that white capital and the state simply moulded and crafted the reserves as they saw fit, while at the same time questioning the idea that African migrants were following in the footsteps of their working-class peers in Europe. Mafeje said that the Marxists and the liberals were so interested in measuring developments in South Africa against the yardstick of Europe than they had failed to appreciate the social logics of uniquely African cultural and political responses to colonialism. He also noted that the committed materialism of the Marxists resulted in them seeing all social change as a response to material conditions.[45]

The persistence of circular migration and continued investment in rural homemaking after apartheid seem to endorse the importance of the socio-cultural arguments around migration.[46] As in many other parts of Africa, and despite the history of industrialisation and the making of a working class, the end of apartheid clearly brought an end to the formal migrant labour system in South Africa—as defined by the labour contracts, the pass laws and the homeland governments. However, it did not shut down the migrant cultures that had entrenched themselves in rural areas over the previous 100 years. In his work on Mexico, Jeffery Cohen argues that the migration debate has been so dominated by economists and demographers that scholars have been reluctant to embrace the idea of different "cultures of migration" which have deep historical roots, cultural significance and social gravity.[47] In the case of South Africa, scholars note the persistence of migrant labour; it was discovered that between 10% and 15% of the working population continued to move between town and country in the way they had previously under apartheid.[48] In this context, it is noteworthy that when Covid-19 hit South Africa between February and June 2020 more than 6 million people physically changed household.[49] The astonishing capacity of people to move from one kinship group to another indicates the existence of multiple webs of social relationships and trans-local connectivity, suggesting that the labour market measure of migrancy is just the tip of the iceberg, hinting at a process of much greater cultural and social significance in the society.

The idea of cultures of migration is a concept that certainly merits much more attention in southern Africa. The concept is different to the idea of migrant culture as it has been conventionally regarded in the South African context. Migrant culture implies a culture that emerges in the townships, shack areas or hostels in the city which is comprised of cultural values, social networks and institutions that actively and deliberately celebrate rural home areas and cultivate the maintenance of migrant ties. Migrant culture is typically contrasted with township culture, which embraces urban consumption and lifestyles, but without necessarily rejecting the rural areas. This urban-rural distinction, emphasised in the literature, does not capture the idea that embracing a culture of migration does not necessarily mean rejecting modernity and globalisation. Indeed, in this sense, it may be argued that there are no longer any migrant cultures in South Africa today, only cultures of migration which connect people across space in culturally complex and diverse ways. To feel connected to a rural home does not mean rejecting modernity, or seeking to be submerged in a pre-colonial ethnic past. It is more a statement of desiring connection to that past and the associated sense of cultural and family identity, while at the same time embracing the new opportunities and identities produced in a democratic South Africa. These bonds were often forged through rituals and the connection of home with rites of passage. When the fear of Covid swept through South Africa in March 2020, many of those who had recently urbanised to cities instinctively thought: should I not go home and be with my family at this time?

In their recent work on post-socialist social change in rural Eastern Europe, Stephen Gudeman and Chris Hann have shown how social and cultural elements of pre-socialist "home base" in rural areas have been reconstituted and reinvented to deal with the stresses of the post-socialistic crisis.[50] In their work they describe a process of social reconstruction where ritual plays a critical role in recovering family unity and loyalties that were pulled apart by socialist collectivisation.[51] In this book we argue that rural communities in South Africa have similarly deployed ritual as a strategy for economic and cultural resilience, survival and reconstruction over the past century in response to colonialism, dispossession and, more recently, neo-liberalism and urbanisation. We argue that after the onset of democracy in South Africa in 1994, circular migration continued in the context of the AIDS pandemic as migrants flooded out of the rural areas only to return home to bury their dead. In the new age of urbanisation, rural homemaking was needed to anchor families against adversity, connect their members to the land of their ancestors, and to care for the sick. These realities allowed family ritual to re-emerge as a formative and foundational force in post-apartheid South Africa. It was both a means of connecting youth and migrants to their homes, and a way of expressing how far families felt they had "progressed" since freedom and democracy. Against this backdrop, this book explores the shock, horror and abiding sense of indignity and alienation associated with the greater "state of exception" imposed in rural areas by Ramaphosa's regime in South Africa from March 2020.

In this book, we focus on Covid and custom in the former Transkei region of South Africa through a culturally informed analysis of political economy, where ritual has played a vital role in shaping the overall response to poverty and external domination.[52] In the next chapter, we show how in the first half of the 20th century, in a context of an enforced migrant labour system and proletarianisation, communities changed their ritual practices to encourage greater cooperation between household and families or wider clan groups. This helped them to increase their resilience and agricultural production and resist colonialism. We suggest that these adaptations were a response to the urgent need for families to lift agrarian production, to defend themselves against being drawn into colonial public works projects and forced migrant labour to the cities. This resilience was broken during apartheid but re-emerged in new forms during heightened urbanisation and the AIDS pandemic; families relied on their rural home as anchors and places of retreat and spiritual security in the heartless world of neo-liberalism and record-breaking unemployment. Based on this analysis, in chapter two we then explore the impact of the Covid lockdown and its assault on ritual and customary practice in rural areas. The chapter reveals the hidden stories behind the state clampdown in these areas and the increasing levels of panic and fear that engulfed families and communities that had been left behind. Chapter three focuses on the medical mayhem that ensued once rural infections rose sharply, placing pressure on a critical weak rural public health system that could not carry the load. The chapter reveals how failures in one area led to problems in others as rural communities were left unprotected and without care, except what they could muster themselves.

The fourth chapter in the book explores the impact of lockdown on rural households and communities, focusing on gender and generational conflicts in households and the parallel pandemic of gender-based violence (GBV). Here we focus specifically on how youth and older women clashed in their struggle for power and resources in the rural areas, and the rising numbers of witchcraft accusations that were implicated in this struggle. Chapter five of the book hones in on the role of local gatekeepers and officials, including police, nurses and traditional leaders, and how they mediated in local affairs and intervened to manage lockdown in various ways. Chapter six deals specifically with the second wave of infection, which started at the end of 2020, and the evidence of cultural resistance—families and communities reclaimed their cultural rights by exhuming bodies that had been buried in plastic without due respect and cultural process, and secretly reburied them. It also explores how rural families reactivated ritual and customs once the lockdown rules fell away. The final chapter reconnects the book to the broader argument about culture and political economy, and the role of ritual in rural life. At the same time, it explores what a post-Covid future might produce in the rural areas, given ruptures the Covid period has brought in ritual life and the diminishing trust and growing disillusionment with the state. Covid has already deepened rural poverty,[53] but could it also bring an end to the interconnections of migrant labour, or will it mark a return to agrarianism and self-reliance in the former homelands?

1

HOMELANDS REMADE

Introduction

This book is centrally concerned with the impacts of Covid-19 regulations and their enforcement on the ritual activities of households and communities in rural South Africa. In this context, this chapter explores how community rituals restructured agrarian social relations in response to colonisation and the advent of the migrant labour system in the eastern parts of the Cape colony at the turn of the 20th century. The chapter places ritual at the centre of local people's struggles to retain autonomy and control over their lives and livelihoods—while needing to pay colonial taxes—and the resistance of proletarianisation after communities were formally incorporated into the Cape colony, and later, the Union of South Africa. The chapter also seeks to introduce the former Transkei region historically and to break down the perception that all "labour reserves" were products of the same histories and may thus be characterised as virtually identical. In the former Transkei, for example, the strong sense of local identity and the function of ritual as a means of social cohesion was a product of the region's relative stability following its colonial capture. Communities and formations of peoples and chieftains were territorialised and settled, sometimes with new neighbours, but also with well-known ones, and consolidated into a formal political system run

33

by magistrates and native commissioners. Between 1955 and 1963 there was nevertheless considerable political upheaval in this area. The apartheid government tried to tamper with traditional authority structures through the Bantu Authorities Act of 1951, attempting to ensure that it had co-opted chiefs to usher in its ethnic national home-land policy.[1] The resistance was dogged and determined in many parts of so-called Transkei territories because of the histories of residential and political stability after colonisation, which the apartheid govern-ment aimed to upend. In this chapter we suggest that strong place-based identities, cultural resistance and the close connections to rural home places in this area were consolidated in the 20th century through neighbourhood beer drinking rituals, male initiation ceremonies and burial rites. We suggest that by the end of the century circular migra-tion, trans-localism and double-rootedness were sustained, even after the migrant labour system was dismantled by the liberation govern-ment after 1994. This occurred as the new democracy was gripped by the AIDS pandemic, primarily due to the need for dignified burial and home-care, supported by social grants—instead of the pursuit of Xhosa masculinity or agricultural self-sufficiency. The concept of trans-localism refers to situations in which developments in different locations connect and influence people at the same time; events in one place, such as a death in the city or the acquisition of a job, have an immediate impact on social relations, livelihoods and belonging in other places. The idea of double-rootedness means that individuals and families feel connected to two places, usually a place of origin and a place of residence.

This chapter thus focuses on the cultural economy of rural home-making before and after apartheid in the former Transkei territories through a cultural economy lens. From this perspective, ritual is seen to occupy a central place in shaping the overall response of rural communities to poverty and external domination. In the first half of the 20th century, resistance to the emerging migrant labour system and proletarianisation was affected through extra-household agrarian solidarities to increase production at home. In this context, neigh-bourhood beer drinking rituals evolved to support the quest for greater self-reliance, especially in areas with good soils and the capac-ity to produce a surplus. The chapter then suggests that increased neighbourliness, activated in response to domination, was consolidated as family-based stick fighting evolved into location-based faction fighting in the segregationist era; tribal authority and territorial citizenship were thus consolidated between the world wars.[2] Faction fighting deepened local territorial identities and greatly elevated the cultural and political importance of male initiation, which was reconstructed through ritual in the rural space.[3] The chapter then turns to the new cultural economy of rural homemaking after democracy in 1994. Increased access to the city produced accelerated outmigration, especially amongst the youth, but also introduced a new era of translocality in an age of social grants, sickness and death during the HIV and AIDS pandemic. Funeral rituals, in which dead bodies were often returned from cities to their rural homes, became a new cultural crucible for the remaking of rural home spaces, in a context of rising suburban nationalism across the country. In other words, these rituals have been influenced by the wider national embrace of sub-urbanism as a form of African nationalism, built on the promises of the ruling party that access to a basic suburban life with modern housing and service for all is the essential definition of South African citizenship. As the cultural forms and meaning of the rural home changed, the focus moved away from agrarianism. New forms of identity politics and social practice marked not the death, but the reconstruction, of the rural home. This sets the scene for the rural Covid crisis of 2020 and the struggle over customary power and practice in the face of a new wave of death and disease.

A patchwork quilt: Colonialism, equivalence and inequality

The Transkei region was colonised by the British between the 1850s and 1894. The primary catalyst for colonisation was the spread of cattle disease in the region, which lead to the great Xhosa cattle killing of 1856–57. Many communities in the western Transkei region burnt their crops and killed their cattle on the recommendation of local chiefs and prophets, who claimed that such action would drive the white colonists into the sea.[4] The prophetic vision that new people would rise from the rivers and the sea to remove the whites and lead an economic, social and moral revival in the indigenous communities did not materialise.[5] Instead, the resulting economic deprivation opened the region to swift, decisive seizure by colonial forces and their allies. In the previous century, the British had colonised the region known as the Ciskei through a series of brutal wars of dispossession; they faced stubborn, determined resistance by Xhosa-speaking peoples.[6] Military victory over the communities in this territory had depended on a divide-and-rule strategy, under which the British colonial government co-opted and deployed Mfecane war refugees, known as the Mfengu or Fingos (meaning wanderers), as well as local Khoi people (known as "Hottentots") to fight the Xhosa chieftains. The British seldom put their own settlers on the front line and often established a buffer zone of Mfengu or Hottentot settlements between the fledgling colonial communities and the frontier beyond, as happened at the Kat River.[7] In the Ciskei region, the long-term aim of the British was to establish a settler colony by extending white sovereignty and settlement across the Eastern Cape from Port Elizabeth to the Kei River.[8] To support this occupation, white settlers were actively encouraged to farm and settle in the region. When the British crossed the Kei River after the 1850s to take control of the so-called Transkei territories—the land between the Cape and the Natal colony to the east—they did not foresee the Transkei becoming settler territory. Rather the main aim was to secure the eastern seaboard of South Africa through annexation and control under a system of indirect rule.[9]

But the British also sought to control the territory by settling large numbers of Mfengu or Fingo in new communities across the Kei River, indicating to local people that they had loyal African allies on their doorstep, who could quickly be mobilised against any uprising. The British made their strategic intent known in the 1850s and 1860s by settling around 50,000 Fingo in villages in the newly created district of Fingoland east of the Kei River.[10] The former residents of this land were either displaced by war or had already scattered because of the Xhosa cattle killing. The British were able to drive the principal chief of the Gceleka people, Chief Sarili, from this territory in the 1850s. With the help of the Mfengu, they then defeated him again in the war of 1867–68 when he tried to return to this land.[11] Mfengu communities and war refugees were also moved into a district known

Map 2: Annexing of the Transkei territories by Britain, 1879–94

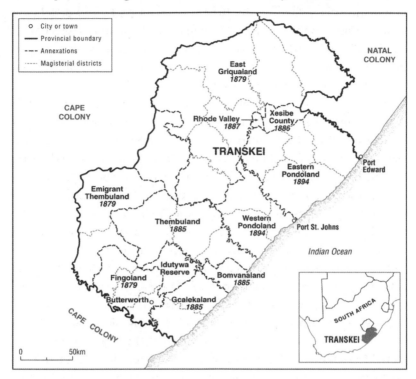

as Emigrant Thembuland in the north-western Transkei. Although the disruptions of colonisation led to social mixing and the realignment of groups, the aim of the British colonial government was not to mix Mfengu with Xhosa (or Gceleka) and other people in the Transkei, but to use them as a threat to any political mobilisation against the state.[12] This pattern of settlement created a patchwork quilt of "red" or "blanket" people, who resisted colonial culture and domination, and new "school" communities from the frontier society in the Ciskei, which was a centre of missionary activity.[13] Many of these, like the Mfengu, had entered as refugees. The creation of new African settlements followed the colonial project across the Transkei, although the greatest density of Mfengu settlement remained based in Fingoland to the west, and thinned to the east, where Mpondo chieftains resided. These territories, known as Pondoland, were

37

finally annexed in 1894.[14] The map below shows how densely the Fingoland was settled by the British with Fingo households being allocated sites on the new location maps, which did not exist for areas outside the new settlement zones. Mission stations were also brought into these new areas, which further marked them off culturally from those that lay beyond their borders.

Although the settlement of the Transkei is more complex than this short summary suggests, the key point here is that, unlike the colonial occupation of the Ciskei territories, the primary aim of the colonial state here was not to eliminate communities through war and create "vacant" territory for white settler occupation and economic improvement; nor was it to actively civilise the local population through education and Christianity.[15] It was rather to incorporate the population that were already there under white domination and colonial rule, without necessarily alienating them from their land or seeking to transform their local production regimes or systems of political authority. The approach adopted in the Transkei was more akin to the indirect rule imposed in British West Africa than the more direct rule imposed in other parts of the Cape and Natal colonies in South Africa in the 19th century.[16] This did not mean that the Transkei was unaffected by the colonial frontier economy into which it had been drawn. Historians like William Beinart have shown that rural communities across the Transkei proved to be highly responsive to the opportunities of the colonial markets in the late 19th century, and quickly adopted new technologies such as the metal disk plough to expand agrarian production for the market.[17] Beinart shows that it was not only the Mfengu or Fingos with mission schooling that could enter the colonial markets; many others who had control over labour and technology could too.[18] Since wagons and metal ploughs were easily purchased by anyone with the money to buy them, the colonial frontier was open for business to all, including non-schooled chiefs and community leaders with land and labour. Beinart shows that the rise of an African peasantry in the late 19th century was not restricted to Africans with colonial cultural capital and formal access to land through registered freehold property.[19]

The American historian Clifton Crais supports this observation of widespread market participation in the former Transkei during the late 19th century, but argues instead that the participation was pre-dominantly caused by the poverty and desperation brought on by war and disruption. He argues that only a small segment of the population—as little as 3%—appears to have been upwardly mobile as a result of market access. The majority, he suggests, entered the market in desperation to sell produce for survival under the traumatic conditions of hunger, conflict and disruption.[20] Notwithstanding the relative virtues of Beinart's rising peasantry argument, and Crais's deepening poverty argument, it seems certain that there was still considerable inequality in wealth amid poverty and hunger in the Transkei territories. Some household heads with large cattle holdings, for example, could aggregate their family wealth through polygamy, creating kinship alliances through marriage. However, the dominant trend across the region from the 1880s was towards smaller households. Scholars argue that the plough made it easier for a surplus to be produced and young men were thus less dependent on staying with their father's kin, if they could get a site of their own to develop. Marriage now became possible at a younger age and homesteads split earlier than before. At the same time, the new agrarianism that accompanied the plough made households more dependent on one another to bring in the crop, as weeding, harvesting and ploughing required inter-household cooperation to meet family subsistence requirements.[21]

Ritual, agrarianism, and territorial cohesion

In the 1960s, the American anthropologist Clifford Geertz wrote about local cultural responses to the colonial dual economy in Indonesia, where large-scale capitalist sugar production coexisted with subsistence production in a traditional rice-producing sector.[22] Geertz described the Javanese peasants as united in their commitment to drive a new cultural economy as a form of adaption under difficult circumstances; this economy was based on social redistribution, innovation and shared poverty. The social system was adjusted to encourage sharing and land use practices changed to accommodate more intensive production on small family rice paddies.[23] In Geertz's view, the traditional sector was trapped by colonialism, but not static. He referred to a process of "agricultural involution", also called "shared poverty", where households collaborated to intensify rice production at the village level to support growing numbers of people on small parcels of land. Geertz saw "involution" as the application of an existing cultural orientation toward "inward elaboration", as seen in Javanese textile and design traditions, to adapt to economic change. Despite criticism from political economists, Geertz insisted that the innovation achieved by the Javanese peasantry under pressure from the colonial economy was essentially culturally informed.

In his extensive work on rural communities in Latin America, Stephen Gudeman makes a structural distinction between the "house economy" of the family and community, which he calls "the base", and the economy of the (capitalist) "corporation" or the hacienda (farm estate), which has a different logic and co-exists in different ways with "the base" in different "culture regions". Gudeman's long-term fieldwork reveals how the house economy logic prioritised life-cycle events, saving, recycling, independence and the repurposing of left-overs (not only food but material items as well), which local people were always trying to defend against external intrusions and domination.[24]

In his analysis of beer drinking rituals in the former Transkei, Pat McAllister[25] elaborates a dual economy strategy like that identified by Geertz in colonial Indonesia and Gudeman in Colombia. The advent of Union in South Africa in 1910 and the implementation of the Land Act in 1913 prevented the expansion and modernisation of the so-called "traditional economies" of the reserves. The state tried to contain the reserves through measures to limit soil erosion and betterment planning. The idea was to ensure that native reserve areas, like the Transkei, could support most of those living there, while also releasing enough migrant labour to drive economic growth at the white-owned mines, industries and farms.[26] Pat McAllister starts his book *Xhosa Beer Drinking Rituals: Power Practice and performance in the South African Rural Periphery* by suggesting that:

> beer drinking rituals ... were very elaborate affairs, highly structured and governed by a complex set of conventions, procedures and customs (*imithetho*), held for a wide variety of significant purposes, accompanied by lengthy debates and discussion as well as by artful oratory.[27]

Following Dietler,[28] McAllister suggests that Xhosa rituals in which beer is shared and consumed are political events: the rituals "act as an instrument and a theatre for political relations", through which "people negotiate relations, pursue economic and political goals, compete for power and reproduce and contest ideological representations of the social order and authority".[29] He claims that the rituals should be seen as "both an instrument of domination and resistance, as an arena for symbolic naturalisation, mystification and contestation of authority".[30] In the first half of the 20th century, plough-driven agrarianism swept through the Transkei while household sizes were shrinking. McAllister argues that cooperative labour was therefore necessary to bring in the maize crop needed to sustain communities. In this context, community-level, work-related redistributive beer drinking proliferated across the region, in both "red" and "school" communities. By the time he encountered these rituals in a "red" community in Shixini on the Transkei coast in the 1970s, they were already in a state of terminal decline in other areas. In this regard, the value of McAllister's book lies partly in its recovery of hidden transcripts of rural resilience and resistance. It reveals what he calls "counter-hegemonic cultural practices" in the Transkei in the early and mid-20th century. McAllister suggests that although beer drinking and ritual activity were already well-known in the Transkei, in the 20th century they were brought together to re-make rural communities and neighbourhoods in the face of colonialism.[31]

Thus, territorial identities were strengthened through agrarian production and regular ritualistic activity which endorsed neighbourhood-based solidarities across the Transkei. They also found expression in the increasing prevalence and popularity of stick-fighting. Sean Redding has observed that the stick-fighting in Transkei in the early 19th century was different to the kind of stick-fighting that became prevalent in the 1930s and 1940s.[32] She suggests that early observers percieved stick-fighting as mainly associated with recreational sparring among boys, often performed during the concluding celebrations in male circumcision rituals.[33] At this time, the region was not at war with colonial forces, stick-fighting activities were not undertaken on a large scale, and they did not generally involve lethal violence. At initiation ceremonies, participants received a knobbed stick and javelin from their relatives and were told that they for protecting the homestead and the local chief. Early observers stated that the heartland of the Xhosa-speaking people was relatively peaceful and that the violence and warfare which later came to define the region were largely absent from rural communities.[34] When South African anthropologist Monica Wilson conducted fieldwork in the Pondoland in the late 1920s, she found that playful stick-fighting was becoming more serious and that there was a "thin line that separated sport from more serious combat".[35] She reported that groups entering an unfamiliar neighbourhood or district without announcing themselves could result in a serious fight between neighbourhood groups, locations and even districts. Noted Xhosa ethnologist J. H. Soga, who also reported on stick-fighting in the Transkei, suggested that serious wounds were now common and that the faction fights were often lethal. South African police reported 1,514 faction fights over a 28-month period between 1929 and 1931, at an average of 54 fights per month, in 27 districts.[36] The faction fights could involve anywhere between a dozen fighters on each side to groups of several hundred combatants.

Like beer drinking, which had played a limited role when Transkei communities were more mobile in the 19th century, stick-fighting had also been a relatively contained community affair for young boys during this period, although both sticks and javelins were carried into war when the chieftaincy or nation was threatened. Redding suggests that stick-fighting transitioned from local sparring to fully-fledged faction fights, where opposing sides were sometimes armed with guns as well as sticks, for more modern reasons—including population pressures and restrictions on access to land. Somewhat surprisingly, Redding does not mention the connection between stick-fighting and beer drinking. South African historian Anne Mager argues that the growing violence, deaths and serious injuries linked with stick fights in the central Transkei were related to migrant labour and the increasing absence of senior men on the mines. This created the space, she argues, for young men to become engaged in expressions of masculinity and conflict that would not have been tolerated when senior men were around to keep the peace.[37] McAllister notes that when things became rowdy at beer drinking rituals, it was usually the senior men who were able to calm things down.[38] However, what both Anne

Mager and Sean Redding seem to overlook is the central role that ritual played in entrenching territorial identities and conflict in the context of land scarcity. By the 1930s and 1940s, Xhosa beer drinking rituals had stabilised and reinforced territorial identities, making stick-fighting both a necessary and inevitable consequence of shared poverty and competition for scarce resources. Like beer drinking, stick-fighting might thus be part of a culturally informed response to colonialism and land scarcity. It bolstered rural production and elevated territorial, neighbourhood identities over kin and clan networks links, which tended to be geographically dispersed. The other critical development in the inter-war years was the rising importance of male initiation, which has been directly linked to the local cultures of faction fighting and migrant labour.[39] Female initiation rites progress fell away during the 20th century as patriarchal power and competition was reenforced through colonialism.[40]

Apartheid planning: Direct rule and rural revolt

While autonomy is important in community formation around rituals, the process of this formation should not be viewed as fully organic, conflict-free and socially coherent. There were many disputes over land and identity across the Transkei territories, especially where Mfengu settlements were imposed in places where local people had long been settled. Many of the faction fights in the Transkei escalated into fights between territorial blocks that had been created in the process of colonial settlement—for example, the continual, violent faction fights that occurred between the inhabitants of mission locations and Mfengu settlements and those living in surrounding Gcaleka communities. The influence of the culture of the mines and the city styles of some migrants also had a profound impact on youth identities and cultural style-making in the countryside.[41] Meanwhile, in areas like Emigrant Thembuland, shrewd traditional leaders, such as local chief Kaiser Matanzima and his family, played clever political games with colonial magistrates and commissioners to extend their political influence over a broad territorial base. Emigrant Thembuland was a mixed area with people from many different sub-ethnic and clan affiliations in the villages, whom Matanzima claimed as his followers.[42] The colonial state agreed to expand the territorial reach of the area under his control in exchange for concessions like the implementation of cattle culling and betterment planning. During the give-and-take of these "homeland" politics at the margins, Matanzima annoyed and frightened hard-working migrants in the city and their families in the villages. They felt he was trading away their possibility of maintaining a rural productive base from which to fight full proletarianisation and poverty.[43] In 1962, groups of migrants from these socially mixed villages who had become embroiled in the politics of the Pan-Africanist Congress (PAC) left Cape Town and returned home to kill Kaiser Matanzima.[44] On disembarking at Queenstown train station, they assaulted and killed two white policemen who wanted to arrest them, and then proceeded on foot over the hills to Matanzima's homestead in Qamata. They were again intercepted and ultimately failed in their attempt on his life.[45]

The case has been well-documented because of the lengthy trial that followed in Queenstown; the threat on white lives posed by the would-be assassins; and the force deployed by the colonial state and the Thembu chief against the communities from which the men came. The authorities brutally suppressed rural uprisings in the Qamata district and across the north-eastern Transkei; these uprisings had been sparked by colonial interventions in agricultural planning and community representation, such as the creation of new tribal authorities.[46] Support was offered to the migrants' struggle by the banned PAC, which promoted the view that South Africa would only be "free in sixty-three" if its followers were prepared to kill whites and remove black collaborators, like Matazima.[47] The unrest in Qamata was linked to the political style and ambition of Kaizer Matanzima, who later became the prime minister of the Transkei homeland; however, it was more specifically related to the regional implications of the 1951 Bantu Authorities Act and the state's promise to implement Ciskei-style "agricultural betterment" in the region. The map below indicates the impacts of the apartheid state's efforts to implement local-level "betterment planning" in the Transkei between 1948 and 1980. In the Ciskei, "betterment" land and settlement planning had affected every community by the mid-1950s, despite the cutting of fences and local resistance in many places.[48] But it is noteworthy that

Map 3: The extent of "betterment" planning in the Transkei, 1980

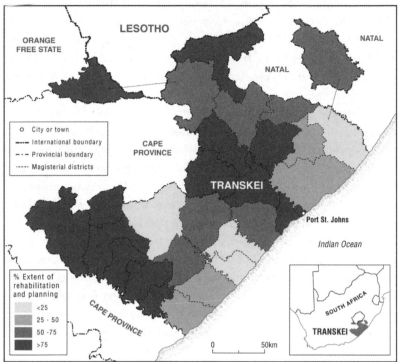

the apartheid state struggled to impose the policy in the Transkei, achieving only limited success along the coast as well as in the central and eastern regions.[49] In this regard, Matanzima's territory of Emigrant Thembuland was quite a densely rehabilitated area, as can been seen in Map 3 above.

In 1960 the state tried to introduced new tribal authority structures, rehabilitation and "betterment" planning in Pondoland, the area located along the coast in the north-east Transkei. This provoked a full-scale rebellion which was only crushed once the army and police were mobilised.[50] Other areas across the region saw continuous political mobilisation and revolt from below. Hand-picked apartheid headmen and chiefs were rejected by communities, who swept the countryside burning collaborators' huts and destroying government equipment and plans related to agricultural "betterment".[51]

Historians and political scientists have debated the role of the liberation movements in political mobilisation in the Transkei in the 1960s. The African National Congress, for example, claimed to be actively involved in the Pondo Revolt against apartheid restructuring in 1960, while the Pan-Africanist Congress claimed to be the prime mover in other areas, especially north-eastern Transkei. There is no doubt that migrants were bringing new ideas and forms of political consciousness into the Transkei during the 1950s and 1960s, stoking the flames of localised resistance. Examples of this include rising anti-white sentiment in the region, following the Pan-Africanist Congress' campaign about the need for a nationalist struggle to end white rule. However, it is also clear that the region's instability during this period was primarily driven by apartheid gerrymandering with tribal authorities and local territorial dispensation. In Pondoland, for example, the catalyst for violence was not anti-white feeling, or even African or pan-nationalist fervour, but rather grievances over appointments of local chiefs and headmen who local people did not support. Groups of dissidents often took to the mountains, creating committees like the co-called i-*kongo* or *makuluspan* groupings. These committees linked up groups across districts and tribal authority areas as resisters mobilised again apartheid restructuring.

The apartheid state suggested that the uprisings were expression of activistic tribalism and were essentially no different from the situation in White Highlands in Kenya, where the Mau Mau groups took "barbaric oaths" in the bushes before "killing whites on farms".[52] The apartheid state used images of white civilisation being overwhelmed by evil African tribalism—driven by the occult, healers and witchcraft—to mobilise white support for a Transkei crackdown using the combined force of the army and the police.[53] The apartheid government exaggerated the threat of regional collapse, while overemphasising the anti-white content of the political protests, to deflect attention from its own programme of hand-picking tribal authorities in the region. In this context, the African nationalism movement and its advocates and intellectuals were naturally eager to reject the narrative of African barbarism and backwardness. Claiming to have organised and orchestrated the revolts was one of the ways in which these movements could challenge the state's narrative. The fear of the Mau

Mau in the white liberal media, which came from a careful tracking of events in Kenya, also played a role in uniting white settler opinion on the need for repressive action in the Transkei. The apartheid state used this fear to force its agenda for ethnic national development. In the early 1960s, Transkei became the first ethnic national homeland to accept self-governance under the new leadership of Kaiser Matazima and his allies. The leadership accepted full political independence as a separate ethnic nation state within South Africa in 1976. Pat McAllister started his fieldwork in the Transkei in 1977, where he observed that many of the region's defining social and cultural practices from the first half of the 20th century were starting to disappear with political restructuring.

But what happened in the Transkei was no simple reversal or linear transition. Under apartheid the region became more integrated into the migrant labour economy. From the 1970s onwards the state wanted to reward the homeland for accepting political independence; it offered rural residents more jobs at the expense of migrants from other regions. There was an influx of population and resettlement in some areas because of the apartheid government's efforts to reverse urbanisation. These interventions coincided with political restructuring, heightened local tensions and territorial fragmentation. However, they did not diminish the spirit of resistance and the quest for rural homemaking within the interstices of racial capitalism and separate development. There was a distinct cultural spirit of defiance and rural resistance in this region, which clung to tradition and custom as a key source of identity and script for social reconstruction. In the former Ciskei in the 1950s and 1960s, the state enforced betterment planning in almost every village and district, mostly against the will of the people. As Map 3 shows, this was far more difficult to achieve in the Transkei, even after the repression of the 1960s. Many rural communities resisted incorporation into the apartheid rural planning rubric and remained defiantly "un-bettered" or "rehabilitated".

Suburban nationalism and trans-locality after democracy

In the 1950s a former Transkei magistrate, H.F. Sampson, described the region as a world of [identical round] "white-faced huts looking

47

down on paths and cattle, on mealie lands without fences, on women at work with their hoes, bare breasted—and over the hill, the chant of young men swinging their way with kerries (sticks) lifted [for fighting]".[54] He writes that while the huts were usually sparsely spread along the coast, denser clusters were also present, especially in locations planned by the colonial government. In the homesteads, women would be stamping mealies with children, with pigs and fowl milling around. Older boys were often herding stock on the hills further away, and parties of men might be viewed on horseback pursuing important business, such as attending a neighbouring beer drinking event.[55] At the same time that Sampson composed this romantic colonial rendition of the traditional Transkei landscape, tourist brochures and postcards were being produced showing picturesque turquoise and white painted huts; images of women in traditional dress smoking long wooden pipes; and men posing in beaded outfits with stick-fighting gear.[56] Elements of this landscape lingered into the 1990s, especially in parts of the Transkei which managed to remain unaffected by government policies promoting "betterment" and closer settlement.

The physical look and feel of the landscape and rural homestead set-up are now different. The older rounds huts and grain storage houses are there but the main house is often designed along suburban lines, as a rectangular dwelling made of new material. Similarly, rural dress styles are no longer markedly different from urban ones, except in small, vanishing segments of the region's older rural culture. The country's main chain stores and fast food companies have opened outlets in the small towns, which have become the local hubs of activity in an almost entirely cash-based rural economy. The changes in the region's consumer and supermarket culture may be described as part of a larger phenomenon of "displaced urbanism",[57] under which the aspirations of rural households have changed as new kinds of freedom and mobility have been experienced since the 1994 introduction of democracy. In this regard, one of the greatest changes for rural people has been the introduction of the right to move and live where they wish, if they can. It took a few years for rapid outmigration to gain momentum among women and youth in the former Transkei. The first wave of outmigration came when the wives of migrants left the countryside to join their husbands in the cities as they moved out of single sex hostels into family housing or informal settlements.[58] This was followed by successive waves of migration among young men and women, who flooded into the big cities looking for work. The Eastern Cape has the highest outmigration rate of any province since the end of apartheid, but it also has large numbers of active migrants who return home regularly. An even larger number of urban Eastern Cape residents plan to retire to their rural homesteads after their urban work careers end.

The complex social and economic disruption and changes that these movements caused in rural communities across the Transkei defy easy explanation. While the evidence shows that the Eastern Cape has lost more people to the large cities than any other province in South Africa, many have not left permanently. The region has seen outmigration but also a shift toward trans-locality for households, which are now stretched across town and country in new ways.[59] Many households have failed to put down roots in urban areas, due to factors including a lack of secure employment and limited land and resources for housing in the cities. This has encouraged families to re-invest in the rural areas where building is cheaper and services can be free. The arrival of big brand stores, basic service provision, fast food outlets and cellphone towers across the countryside has allowed migrants, who originally left for the bright lights and modern services of the city, to re-evaluate their investment and retirement strategies. For others, permanent urbanisation was never an option, and it was only ever about choosing the right moment for a rural return. At the same time, there are many who want to put down roots in the big cities and ensure that their children receive a decent education and access better opportunities for the future, uncompromised by the rurality of their parents' generation. Much has changed—most of all, perhaps, regional perceptions of the importance of agricultural production and rituals which reinforce local-level cooperation and sharing.

The changing cultural and social orientation in the rural Transkei over the past two decades is not just the result of shifts in mobility and economic opportunity. They have been influenced by the wider national embrace of sub-urbanism, built on the the ruling party's promise that access to a basic suburban life with modern housing and service for all is the essential definition of South African citizenship. Together with the development of mall and shopping centres across the country, this has fuelled consumer culture and shifted the focus away from production, including in the rural areas. This shift to an ideology of consumption and sub-urbanism, especially amongst the younger and middle generations, has diminished the involvement of rural households in agrarian pursuit. These days rural household would prefer to be in a position to buy things from the supermarket rather than grow them. However, high levels of unemployment, poverty and food insecurity do make many rural households dependent on garden produce for survival. This situation has been aggravated by the impact of Covid and the loss of jobs associated with the pandemic.[60]

Ritual life in the time of HIV and AIDS

As rural lives, freedoms and aspirations changed with the introduction of democracy, South Africa simultaneously became the global centre of the HIV and AIDS pandemic.[61] Women and youths were the foremost victims of this disease, which ravaged urban areas and informal settlements. The South African government rejected the science on HIV and AIDS as Eurocentric; its denialism exacerbated the harm caused by the pandemic, as the official stance was a refusal to acquire and distribute medications that might have reduced the death toll.[62] By the end of the 1990s, 52% of all deaths in South Africa were HIV and AIDS related, many of them involving young men and women who often died shortly after being infected.[63] At the time, doctors in Eastern Cape hospitals said the death toll in the region was at least double that indicated by the official figures.[64] Rural villages and settlements which had until then been the sites of a population exodus were brought back to life; ill young men and women returned for the support of their mothers and grandmothers, who were now receiving monthly government pensions and could care for them before they died. The literature is replete with harrowing accounts of how the pandemic destroyed the hopes and dreams of a new generation of urbanising youth, replacing them with a nightmare of rural retreat, illness and death.[65]

In the process of this tragic transition, rural ritual life regenerated on a major scale. Funerals were organised almost every weekend across the region to bury the victims of the HIV and AIDS pandemic.[66] During apartheid, the white state and funeral houses had tried to manage the death industry in the city, ensuring that black bodies travelled to registered city cemeteries and hygienic burial practices were adopted. After apartheid, black-owned funeral parlours came to dominate the sector; their owners were the second most successful township entrepreneurs after taxi owners.[67] The HIV and AIDS era was also a time when the funeral industry boomed in townships. The shuttling of bodies and mourning between town and countryside was commonplace. Family members who grew too sick to cope in the cities made their way home to die. This placed considerable burden on rural kin, especially the aged who were forced to bear responsibility for financial support and home-based care.[68] Others never made it home, and died in the city, where they were sometimes also buried. Most often, however, every effort was made by the family to ensure that the bodies were transported home for burial.

Research undertaken in Pondoland, where the non-profit organisations Doctors without Borders (Médicins Sans Frontières) and the Treatment Action Campaign set up a base, found that many young women had returned to die.[69] Before becoming ill, many of them had lost contact with their rural homes after starting a new life in Durban The strain that this return migration placed on already poor rural households has still not been fully documented and appreciated. The number of HIV and AIDS orphans absorbed into the homes of grandparents, neighbours and kin in the rural areas also remains greatly under-estimated; it is only partially visible in the massive regional demand for foster-care grants. Despite the hidden costs and strains of the pandemic on rural households, a change in state policy did lead to the increased availability of anti-retroviral treatments at rural clinics, making a significant difference to how the disease could be managed in both urban and rural areas.[70] Nevertheless, it is fair to say that urban and rural black South African households have been living with death every day since the end of apartheid, and have constantly reflected on ways of dying and burying the dead.[71] Throughout this, women, especially older women, bore the brunt of the culture of care that was needed to nurse their sick sons and daughters and make the preparations for death and burial. Many women invested in local social networks, informal savings clubs and burial societies so that they could provide dignified funerals in the rural areas.

In the early 2000s, the anthropologist Andrew Ainslie collected records on 100 rituals in the former Ciskei. He discovered that there was little emphasis on neighbourly household cooperation in these rituals; most of them were managed by rural matriarchs or other women and designed to promote the status and standing of specific families and households in the wider community. This shift from neighbourhood solidarity to family status and reputation has also become a dominant feature of ritual in the Transkei. Part of the reason for this is that funerals are inherently family affairs; they map the life trajectories of those who have died, reflecting on what they achieved and contributed to their families and the community. The family will host the funeral ritual at which the deceased is celebrated before burying them. Burial is a family matter which takes place at home in the rural areas, often in the yard at the homestead. In the democratic era and since the advent of HIV and AIDS, one of the most striking features of funerals in poor black communities has been their escalating cost. A large survey undertaken in rural areas showed that families were now seemingly competing with one another in hosting funerals, to show how much they could afford to spend on the burial rites of family members.[72] In KwaZulu-Natal it was estimated, based on a sample of over 25,000 cases, that the cost of rural funerals often exceeded the annual income of the households concerned.[73] The rising costs were in part made possible due to the extension of credit to black families. There were also new forms of insurance created by the financial industry in the context of HIV and AIDS.[74]

Given the private and family focus of rural funerals, it would be inappropriate to suggest that these represent large public or political events—such as those held in the cities during the struggle against apartheid, when permission to gather to bury the dead was used in a direct challenge to the state to create mass meetings that would otherwise have been outlawed.[75] In this context, public funerals were choreographed as performative events designed to have a direct political impact. By contrast, ordinary rural burials were seldom staged in ways that deliberately challenged local political leaders or traditional authorities. However, they did project family identities and values within the rural setting. It is in this context that the competitive ethos of conspicuous consumption and ostentation came to play a role after the end of apartheid; rural families tried to illustrate to their neighbours on ritual occasions how far they had progressed away from the old rural lifestyles.

In a trans-local culture of death, urbanising families were constantly returning to rural areas for funerals, spending many hours with relatives in taxis and then being reunited with the rural family in the countryside. Funerals therefore became very influential in the urbanisation of rural homesteads after the introduction of democracy in 1994, and particularly at the height of the HIV and AIDS pandemic. In the first half of the 20th century, McAllister and other scholars showed how the "public sphere" at community rituals and beer drinking reinforced family loyalties, gender and generational hierarchies and, critically, neighbourhood cooperation in agricultural production. In the early 21st century, these rituals played a similar role as deaths caused by the HIV and AIDS pandemic brought families back together at home to re-evaluate their life projects and family identities. This new trans-locality had a profound impact on the Transkei countryside. From around 2000 it was accompanied by great investment in rebuilding rural homesteads, remodelling them in the image of suburban citizenship.[76] The primary investment in the re-imagined rural homestead was provided by the younger generation, especially women, who had migrated to the cities. Many of them no longer conceived their futures as their parents and grandparents had, yet they still remained connected to their places of origins and family homes.

In urban fieldwork conducted in Cape Town, many youths said that the present possibility of death and funeral cycles which entailed moving between town and countryside had fundamental implications for their social lives and aspirations in the city. Many were fatalistic about death and dying because they viewed it as such a common occurrence. At the same time, mutuality with families in cities was being reconstituted around a moral economy of death, and the obligation of families to ensure that their dead were taken back home for a dignified burial and smooth passage into the afterlife among their ancestors. The indignity of urban life under conditions of poverty made the dignity of returning home to be laid to rest seem particularly desirable. It is a similar sense of cultural purity and dignity that has encouraged so many African families to rebuild their family homesteads in the countryside since the end of apartheid. As Bank has shown, younger working women in the cities are often the leading figures in this quest for rural reconstruction and the preparations for retirement and retreat.[77]

Conclusion

The broad aim of this chapter has been to draw attention to the fundamental role of ritual in the colonial Transkei, not as a remnant of pre-colonial cultural forms dragged into the modern world because of the incapacity of rural people to accept and respond to change, but rather as a vector for social change, cultural reconstruction and resistance. The chapter highlights how a new kind of beer drinking emerged across the Transkei after colonisation, allowing communities to make maximum use of new agricultural technologies and consolidate community-level strategies of resistance to proletarianisation and external domination. The emergence of new beer drinking rituals helped neighbours to acknowledge the need for place-based mutual interdependence as they became partners in reshaping the patterns of rural production. This generated a surplus to brew beer and socialise, as well as the maize that fed their families and supported their capacity to resist external domination. The ubiquity and intensity of these ritual activities across the Transkei had a profound impact on territorial identity formation and faction fighting in the pre-apartheid period. The tradition of stick-fighting had occurred on a much smaller scale in the pre-colonial era, but in the early and mid-20th century it escalated and evolved into larger-scale faction fights, in the context of land scarcity and the consolidation of sedentary territorial communities.

With apartheid restructuring, the state required the ethnic homelands to be directly and instrumentally functional to white domination and capital accumulation. In the Transkei, this required much more intervention than had been undertaken during the segregationist era. The apartheid government suddenly imposed restructured tribal authorities and pushed the agenda of agricultural "betterment", similar to the agenda implemented in the former Ciskei, where virtually every community had been resettled and refashioned by the state's agricultural officials. The tradition of silent resistance was rapidly transformed into open revolt across the entire region during the 1950s and into the 1960s. The high-water mark of the rural revolts was the Pondoland revolt of 1960, which followed the Sharpeville massacre and Langa uprisings of March 1960. Evidence from the region suggests that local communities were far more concerned about apartheid interventions in land allocations and tribal authority systems than they were in ridding the areas of white officials and traders. The Commission of Inquiry into the Pondo Revolt of 1960, for example, found that some local white traders supported and armed the rebels; the bonds of trust between local whites and black residents seem to have broken after rather than before the revolt. In retrospect, it appears that the apartheid state escalated the racial dimension of the Transkei violence to win settler support for a decisive campaign of repression and political restructuring, and ultimately usher in homeland self-government. Transkei became the first independent ethnic national state in South Africa in 1976.

After the introduction of democracy in 1994, a suite of government policies and a new Constitution affirmed the right of all South Africans to urban housing. Massive official efforts to relocate poor residents from places like the Transkei to new public housing schemes in the city were launched. Outmigration from the Transkei soon accelerated to such an extent that it became a leading sending area for cities like Cape Town, Durban and Johannesburg. At the same time, the roll-out of the infrastructure for pensions across the Transkei brought some financial security to rural households who no longer received regular remittances from absent migrants, many of whom were seeking work.[78] Home-sickness and death in the form of the HIV and AIDS pandemic stalked the new democratic generation wherever they went and reconstituted kinship and migration patterns in significant ways. Without effective urban healthcare and with the need to bury the dead in their rural homes, the social fabric of migrant life and trans-locality had to be reconstituted. The simultaneous arrival of freedom, urbanisation and citizenship, together with the need to reconstitute family relations in the rural home space in the face of HIV and AIDS, helped to dissolve older forms of ideological and cultural resistance and produce new ones. The old contrast between the rural and the urban started to fall away, as ideas of citizenship and belonging swept through rural home spaces and social relations.

2

DEATH AND NAKED LIFE

Hospitals, on the one hand, are powerful for saving lives; but as places to die they are amoral, dangerous and devoid of ceremonial history and haunted by spirits. Houses, on the other hand, are optimal for dying because they are infused with moral power, a history of beneficial ceremony and family living.

The Spirit Ambulance: Choreographing the End of Life in Thailand,
by Scott Stonington, © 2020 by Scott Stonington.
Published by the University of California Press.

Introduction

In rural South Africa, funerals are family and community affairs. They are not usually managed by the state, funeral directors, local government officials or hospital staff. They are not occasions at which one expects to find policemen, health officials and funeral directors dictating proceedings and behaviour, or threatening arrests and fines. Families and religious leaders are normally given relative freedom to bury the dead in dignified ways, according to tradition and religious belief. However, as Covid-19 spread through the country, funerals and other customary practices, including male initiation rites, were identified as high-risk sites of infection, especially in rural areas where a disproportionately large number of these rituals occurred.[1] Since the 1990s, South Africa's increasing urbanisation has resulted in more people being buried in the cities; during the Covid crisis this led to urban graveyards filling past their capacity. However, many families, especially first-generation immigrants, still maintain a strong tendency to bury family members at their rural homesteads. These practices were entrenched during the HIV and AIDS pandemic, when many sick family members would return to their rural homes to die. From Cape Town and the Western Cape hundreds of bodies return to homesteads in the Eastern Cape for burial every weekend. The same pattern is also evident in Johannesburg and Gauteng where the dead are redistributed to their rural homes in every corner of the country (and the continent) through a national network of combi taxi, burial societies and funeral services. Family and relatives follow the bodies home where they mingle with relatives and neighbours before returning to the city. This process often takes a weekend; mourners leave the cities by midday Friday arrive at their rural home in the middle of the night or early on Saturday morning, and then leave again by Sunday midday to ensure that they can be back at work on Monday. Those without regular jobs might stay longer to help out at home.[2]

With the declaration of a State of Disaster in South Africa in March 2020, funerals were immediately viewed by the state as potential "super spreader" events which needed tight management, control and monitoring. The regulations for funerals produced in April 2020 sought, among other things, to restrict travel between provinces; control interaction with Covid-19 infected bodies; enforce sanitising and physical distancing; restrict attendance at funerals; shorten rituals; and limit the collective consumption of food and alcohol at these events. In addition to these measures, large rural customary practices and gatherings were also banned during lockdown.[3] In the gap between cultural observance and statecraft, customary practices and funerals immediately became major targets for law enforcement in the fight against Covid-19 in rural South Africa. The assumption seemed to be that both rural communities and mourners from the city were likely to ignore state regulations in the seclusion of their rural homes. The state therefore needed to show, in no uncertain terms, that it meant business when it came to containing the spread of Covid-19. To demonstrate their commitment to implementing the Covid-19 regulations, the police force swept across the Eastern Cape region during March and April, disrupting funerals and closing down customary gatherings, especially initiation schools. Where they found gatherings of more than 50 people at funerals, situations where social distancing was not observed, or where food and beer were obviously being consumed communally, the police tipped over drums of traditional beer and pots of food and sent people home.[4] The police were also seen closing down initiation schools in Nxarhuni village near East London and in various places around King William's Town, while they recalled initiates from "the bush" in Libode, Ngqeleni, and areas east of Mthatha.[5] It was reported that there were over 100,000 arrests made in the rural Eastern Cape and other parts of South Africa during this period.[6]

The repressive state and police response to the threat of Covid-19 in rural areas created a culture of fear in these communities. In June and July 2020 this culture of fear was entrenched when many rural clinics and hospitals were forced to shut down at the height of infections due to lack of Personal Protective Equipment (PPE), absence of deep cleaning protocols and the rapid increase in infections. Communities in the rural Eastern Cape often spoke about the Covid-19 period as one where the state "closed the gate" (*ukuvala isango*) on them, shutting them out and bullying them at a time of great fear and uncertainty.[7] They claimed that rural families were disrespected and treated as ignorant and deviant, rather than part of any solution or strategy to mitigate the spread of the virus. They also stated that they were assumed to be socially unresponsive and culturally conservative when they were constantly dealing with change and transformation.

Some recalled how they had to manage the HIV and AIDS pandemic in the 1990s and early 2000s areas when there was little state support and widespread denialism. They remembered the hope they felt when Médicins Sans Frontières arrived in the Eastern Cape and actively engaged communities on key issues, from disclosure to disease management. In the end, however, after the state stopped supporting AIDS denialism it opted for a bio-medical approach by distributing anti-retroviral pills, rather than adopting a more holistic approach to care and engagement.[8]

Rural families were shocked by the intensified state efforts to control death rites and funeral practices as the pandemic worsened in South Africa over June and July 2020. Fear and panic first intensified with the police raids and intensified regulation in March and April. Opportunities for community engagement were then lost as tighter controls and restrictions on funeral attendance and the management of dead bodies were imposed with increasing harshness. By the time infections peaked at the end of July 2020, rural communities across the Eastern Cape were literally in a state of panic about the increasing numbers of "improper funerals" that were ending in chaos and confusion. They were not only angered by the state violence of the police's actions at rural funerals, but were also confused and disorientated by the measures imposed on families, which they felt undermined the spiritual integrity and cultural dignity of the rituals. These measures included denying the family a chance to wash and dress the body, the wrapping of bodies in multiple layers of plastic so the deceased was barely visible, and the shortening and restricting of ceremonies that undermined the performance of "proper" cultural rites. This chapter shows how the regulations created anxiety, fear and spiritual insecurity in communities, not only because of the way they were implemented by the state through the police, but because they made it difficult for families to feel a sense of spiritual and social closure after Covid funerals. The growth in the size and significance of family funerals in the rural Eastern Cape meant that the crackdown on these ritual and social events came as a shock. Instructed by the state, the police and funeral parlours struck at the social core of rural life and belief in South Africa.

In terms of the book's theoretical framing, this chapter seeks to illustrate how the imposition of a greater state of exception in the rural areas created a situation where Agamben's idea of the bare life—where mere survival was all that rural people expected after apartheid—became a naked life, stripped of dignity, spiritual security and the possibility of meaningful social reproduction. The chapter focuses both on the way rural funerals have been changing in recent times, especially in the context of AIDS, and how the state's repressive Covid regime created a climate of fear, anxiety and anger in rural areas, as families buried their loved ones without dignity, certainty and spiritual security. The chapter demonstrates how the state prioritised shutting down rural customary call in the national police clampdown and used rural funerals throughout 2020 to generate fear and compliance. "Traditional" rural ritual was painted as a "super spreader"—an extreme case of pathological practice that could create the country's "worst nightmare". Constant references to individual funerals in the Eastern Cape in particular—like the one at Machibini in the Port St. Johns area of the former Transkei—was a constant theme in the discourse of the state and the suburban media. The chapter also shows why the wrapping of bodies in plastic created such hysteria in rural areas, as it challenged the very foundation of cultural survival and social reproduction. The focus of the discussion is specifically on the impact of the first wave of infections between April and July 2020.

Death, modesty and mourning

In South Africa, dead bodies are often viewed as spiritually unstable and dangerous because they are in a liminal state as the spirit moves between the world of the living to an ancestral afterlife.[9] If this transition is not carefully managed through communication and ritual treatment, and the body disposed of quickly, then there is always the chance that the spirit can be captured by evil or malevolent forces. The social anthropologist Monica Wilson (née Hunter), who worked among the Mpondo people in the former Transkei in the 1920s, noted that family members would start to wail as soon as a death had taken place in the homestead or *umzi*.[10] The family would carry the dead body outside the door of the hut and wrap it in a blanket (or formerly in skins). Every effort would then be made to bury the dead as quickly as possible after death because the "corpse is regarded as contaminating and dangerous".[11] In those days, communities throughout this region used to bury the dead in a crouched position, but after missionary influence became widespread the dead were also often buried in coffins lying down.[12] Some of the deceased's valued possessions were also buried with the coffin, such as beads, spearheads, blanket pins or knives; it was believed the deceased would need these items as they carried on their lives as ancestors (*amathongo*) in the next world. Maize, pumpkin seeds and husks were also sometimes added to the mix of dirt and thorns used to fill the grave. The thorns were included to protect the body from the work of witches, which could torment the spirit and bring bad luck to the family.[13]

When the male head of the *umzi* died, it was the responsibility of the eldest son to bury his father. If the son was not available, then the next most senior male kin took over the duty. A small group of male kin usually engaged with the body and spoke to the corpse while it was washed, cleaned, and dressed by female kin; it was then taken from the hut to the burial site next to a *kraal*.[14] All immediate family members were normally buried between the *kraal* and the main house, with the most senior men close to the *kraal*. Those who had been disloyal to the family, were associated with witchcraft, or had died violently were buried on the far side of the *kraal* facing away from the *umzi*. Pregnant women or women breastfeeding babies would not be allowed near the corpse; women in general were kept away from the body. After the burial everyone in the *umzi* would go to the river to wash before returning to the homestead where a beast would be slaughtered. The gravediggers and others who had been close to the body would take the added precaution of washing their hands in the liquid from the animal's gall bladder. The slaughtered animal would then be prepared for eating; neighbours would also eat this "beast of washing" (*nkomo yokuhlambo*).[15]

During the period of the burial, the immediate family often did not leave the homestead. Milk was spilt on the ground to ward off danger and no man was meant to sleep with his wife. The men and children also often shaved their heads. After three or four days, beer was typically made or a goat killed to "wash the mouth". Only those who had washed, including with special medicines, were safe to interact socially with non-family members. The ritual process steered the members of the immediate family away from the threat of pollution and danger presented at death into a phase of mourning. Before the process of mourning began the blankets and clothes of the deceased were burnt. The widow had to ensure that all traces of the husband were erased from the homestead before engaging in a prolonged period of mourning, often longer than a year. Within six months to three years, a second beast was slaughtered in a ceremony known as *ukubuyiswa* (bringing the spirit home), to help the deceased take their place among the ancestors and to make it easy for them to return to the homestead. This was not the beast of "washing" to ward off danger, but one of social integration and stabilisation. The ceremony brought together family, neighbours and extended kin. In the 1920s and early 1930s, Monica Wilson suggested that the Pondo, like other Xhosa-speaking people generally in the Eastern Cape:

> have a great distaste for speaking of anything connected to death. The name of a person who has recently died is never mentioned in conversation. Children are warned not to mention people that have died and that it is ill-mannered to introduce the subject of death into any conversation ... Christians tell me that the pagan fear of the corpse, and distaste for speaking of death, is not so great as formerly, their attitudes have been modified by the attitudes of Christians.[16]

While Xhosa and Pondo customs traditionally differed in some respects—for example, around the issue of male initiation—their approach to death and burials was very similar. The accounts of funerals in this region from anthropological, local and mission accounts suggest that, besides the fear of pollution, potential witchcraft and misfortune, these occasions were modest affairs. They brought together local people, neighbours and kin in a process that laid the deceased to rest within the grounds of the homestead and started a prolonged process of mourning and observance until the spirit could return to the homestead.

The contemporary Xhosa writer, Siphe Potelwa[17] suggests that family and community cooperation were always vital when managing death within the spirit of *ubuntu* (humanity), where *umtu ngumtu ngabantu* (a person is a person because of other people). He claims that in the rural parts of the former Transkei where he grew up, death invoked a spirit of cooperation and care; this is expressed in the concept of '*ndwandwe*', which meant a form of cooperation amongst women, where they simply came together to assist each other. He says this is similar to the practice of "*ilima*", where men, women and children come together to assist in the weeding or harvesting of the land. He argues that the original burial societies in the region were an extension of this spirit; they also connected people from the same rural localities across town and country. In the case of his own life,

Potelwa recalls how this spirit of cooperation was invoked when his father died shortly after the transition to democracy. He remembers the modesty of the ritual and the extended period of mourning:

> After my father's death, my mother wore black clothes, and my siblings and I had our hair shaved. We wore buttons which were covered in black cloth. All these rituals lasted for a period of one year, after which the *ukubuyiswa* ceremony took place where an ox was slaughtered, and our father's clothes were distributed as a token of remembrance, first amongst the children and then amongst the extended family.... Prior to the distribution of my father's clothes, a ritual was performed in which a portion of the bile juice and blood from the slaughtered ox was mixed with water and sprinkled with the branch of a tree over the clothes. The ceremony was marked by happiness, and, for the first time we were allowed to make jokes about my father, something that had not be allowed during the year-long mourning.

Colonial conquest came to the former Transkei in the latter half of the 19th century. Communities were placed under colonial rule but not necessarily relocated or resettled, as we explained in the first chapter. This was not the case in Ciskei territories to the west, which had been forged out of war, as well as other parts of the former Transkei. In these areas, families were moved around and family graves scattered. It was often necessary over time to rebury kin through a process called "fetching the spirit" or *ukulanda amaxhego* (fetching the ancestors), resettling them closer to the new family homes. Phila Dyantje from the former Ciskei explained that his family and clan had their spiritual heartland in the Amatola mountains, but they were resettled by the colonial government in the Amatola basin.[18] Phila's family decided not to disturb the ancestors' graves, and instead returned to their old spiritual sanctuary in the mountains to perform rituals and bury family members. By connecting their current place of residence to the grave sites through regular rituals, communication with the ancestors was maintained.

Chris De Wet and Erik Mgujulwa, scholars of forced removals in the Ciskei under apartheid, have illustrated how ritual practices and burial rites were adapted in conditions of forced removal to fetch the ancestors and bring scattered kin together in a new place of residence.[19] The process, they explain, was often initiated by reoccurring dreams that related family misfortunes or hardship to the scattering of ancestors and family disunity, often exacerbated by histories of migrant labour. Resolving these issues was complex, especially fetching the ancestors and introducing them to the new place of dwelling; family members had to agree on adjustments to ritual. In their ethnography of the process of fetching, De Wet and Mgujulwa show that there has been constant adaption and innovation that involves both "continuity and change".[20]

The issues discussed above are common in South Africa, as resettlement and forced removal have been a critical part of the colonial experience. There are relative few areas in the former homelands where residential patterns have been as settled as the former Transkei.[21] In her work in the former Lebowa homeland beyond Johannesburg, for example, Deborah James has shown how home funerals and burials rites entrench family claims to land and territory, in a country defined by colonial dispossession.[22]

In the current age of urbanisation, the question of fetching the spirit is most often related to ensuring that the deceased can be safely transported from an urban mortuary to their rural homestead. This often involves collecting the body from the mortuary and returning it first to the place of residence in the city where relatives and friends can bid their personal farewells. The corpse is then transported to the rural Eastern Cape for burial. Given that dead bodies are spiritually vulnerable, it is necessary for close relatives to accompany the body and watch over it on the journey home. In the post-apartheid period, a whole range of new services were developed by entrepreneurs in the townships; they promised to help families with "spiriting" their loved ones home and ensure that the whole funeral process went as smoothly as possible. Dignity here was often associated with extravagance. The cost and character of rural funerals changed after apartheid, as many additions, innovations and adjustments were made through the new "burial industry".

Spirit taxis, migrancy and rural modernity

In his book *The Spirit Ambulance*, Scott D. Stonington contrasts local perceptions of death and dying in hospital and at home in Buddhist communities in northern Thailand.[23] Buddhists believe in reincarnation, in much the same way that many Africans believe the dead are reborn as ancestors, who continue to influence the lives of their families after death. In the Eastern Cape it is believed that very old people make the transition to becoming ancestors (*amathongo*) even before they die.[24] The spiritual transition from this world to the next is not an event but a process, which has to be managed socially and ritually. The deceased must move from a state of impurity or contagion to a state of ritual purity and harmony with the spirit world. The process is guided by the living, through attention to ritual preparation and internment of the body. In addition, to ensure the safe passage to the other world, the close kin or survivors of the deceased need to ensure that the social disintegration occasioned by death is repaired. They must ultimately re-integrate back into the community and group solidarity must be preserved. Both of the above transitions are connected. Death rites and the funeral process serve to guide both the deceased and the living safely into a "beneficial and life-giving balance with each other".[25] In Africa and Thailand, as well as many other parts of the world, it is believed that the quality of one's rebirth, reincarnation or afterlife is affected by the conditions under which one leaves the world of the living, and how one is ushered into the new world by those who are left behind. This is precisely why many Thai Buddhists want to die at home, where they feel comfortable, cared for and have developed a strong sense of belonging through life.[26]

Stonington uses the term "spirit ambulances" to refer to the vehicles that carry dying patients from urban hospitals in Thailand to their homes, so that they can die in peace with their spirit at rest.[27] This belief that dying at home is better than dying in a hospital or in the city, is widely embraced in South African cities too, but not everyone manages to get home before dying. This was especially true during the HIV and AIDS pandemic. Rebekah Lee, who conducted fieldwork on Cape Town funerals between 2008 and 2010, noted how much the funeral industry had changed in the city since post-apartheid deregulation.[28] New African entrepreneurs, especially taxi owners, entered the market with a wide variety of products to jazz up their "spirit taxis", which ferried bodies and mourners seamlessly between town and countryside. Lee documents how the new funeral and taxi businesses offered a range of products including embalming services to preserve bodies, expensive coffins and additional extras including fake lawns and carpets, as well as entertainment and refreshments for city mourners before their departure.[29] The changes in the funeral business and the commodification of services were supported by the continuities in circular migration and double-rootedness.[30] The HIV and AIDS pandemic was a factor in the constant shuttling of people and bodies between urban and rural areas, but the congested living conditions, informal housing and insecure employment in the cities also contributed to the processes of rural reconnection, or "displaced urbanism".[31] In his 1995 novel *Ways of Dying*, Zakes Mda tells the story of an itinerant urban youth who makes his living as a professional mourner in the time of AIDS, moving from one funeral to the next. The mourner meets a kindred spirit from his rural home area, and they move in together in a shack. The interior walls of the shack are then plastered with magazine pictures of perfect modern kitchens, bedrooms and lounges, as they escape the grimness and pain of urban life in suburban fantasies that are seemingly impossible to realise. In post-apartheid South Africa, the urban poor often continue to see possibility and promise in building for their families at home, while waiting for the state to delivery houses and services in the city—or enough money to raise a bond.[32]

Researchers on funerals in the time of Covid in the Transkei have commented on how family spending on funerals in rural areas has increased exponentially over the past decade. Insurance products, taxi services and burial societies now provide the products that families need to celebrate the status of their family. Families aim to outdo each other in terms of the size and scale of funeral events, with fancy coffins, costly tombstones, elaborate programme design, meals both before and after the burial and even video equipment. Not everyone can afford these luxuries and extras, but a trend towards competitive ostentation has become embedded in a social and cultural landscape that was previously defined by modesty and communalism. The traditional earlier desire to bury as soon as possible after death has also apparently been replaced by a long process of ritual extension that can last weeks; bodies were sometimes kept on ice while final arrangements were made for the funeral. The pressure to push up the costs often came from family members in the cities as much as it did from those back home. The consequences of these shifts were already evident in the early 2000s.

A major quantitative survey of data collected between 2003 and 2005, and involving more than 20,000 households in KwaZulu-Natal, showed that funeral expenses rose sharply after apartheid: "households are expected to spend a third of their annual income on funerals (in the year of the death), an amount shaded up or down according to status".[33] A Soweto household income survey at the same time discovered that families were choosing funerals that cost between three to five times their household monthly income. In another study in Johannesburg, Veni Naidu found that low-income families were spending on average just under R10,000 on the funeral expenses of a single family, which did not include additional costs on food, transport and other frills.[34] In his writing, Siphe Potelwa contrasts how different his mother's funeral in the 2000s was from his father's in the 1990s. He explained that by the time his mother died in the 2010s, his family had fallen victim to the presence of conspicuous consumption and the politics of display in the matter of funerals. While personally well-aware of this trap, Potelwa was ultimately unable to prevent the costs from spiralling out of hand because his family wanted "the best" for his mother. He noted that the purpose of funerals seemed to have shifted from rituals that reflected the value of modesty and mourning, to ones that celebrated the life of the deceased and the status of the family. In this sense, they appeared more after mourning bringing back the spirit events, which are also sometimes called "after tears", than the actual funerals of old. Potelwa blamed himself for the being duped by the tricks of consumerism, or what he called "bastardised Westernisation", without fully recognising how much rural society in the former Transkei had changed since the 2000s.[35]

These developments are, of course, not unique to South Africa. In many parts of the continent today, upwardly mobile migrant families try to outdo each other with ostentatious displays of wealth at family rituals, including funerals. In Ghana, fantasy coffins are sold on the internet at huge prices, some in the shape of cell phones which are said to keep the line open to heaven. Stylised home video productions of the rituals are circulated and stored as mementos of family unity, modernity and progress. In South Africa, funeral parlours offer embalming services or refrigerated transport home for the deceased, as well as double-decker buses for mourners. Portable green lawns create a particular middle-class, suburban pathos at some funerals.[36] While noting all these changes, Lee and Vaughan warn that it is tempting to argue that this kind of commodification empties these rituals of their spiritual and social content, marking a "great transformation in African death cultures".[37] This would be a gross oversimplification, they insist, because burials in Africa have always been about status and wealth, as much as they have also expressed social connectedness, embeddedness and belonging. They also argue that money and commercial transactions cannot always be easily separated from local belief systems, sociality and exchange. Indeed, commodities are malleable mediators in local cultures and not simply markers of Western capitalist consumption, as is sometimes assumed.[38] The connection in South African between ostentatious funerals and the desire of families to project themselves as upwardly mobile and modern is plain to see, but this certainly does not imply these rituals have lost meaning or significance. Quite the opposite, it would appear, as they are now asked to carry such a huge cultural and symbolic load at a time of transition.

In our fieldwork during the Covid-19 pandemic we found that some of our respondents applauded the government for imposing stricter rules that cut the costs of funerals, such as not allowing dead bodies to linger as expenses escalated. A shortening of the ceremonial events, we were told, would benefit everyone because it would reduce fruitless costs. Less food could be served and less ostentation would be invited. At our discussions, traditional leaders in the Eastern Cape also commented on the need to cut down on the cost of funerals, saying that rural families were suffering because they spent so much on funerals. Media and academic commentators also suggested that the shock treatment of the new regulations might bring people to their senses in an industry that was "out of control". One informant said that funerals only brought "tears", and that there were no more "after tears" celebrations to be had because of the crippling costs of funerals for rural people.[39]

But, despite the widespread perception that the cost and commodification of funeral rites had gone too far in the Transkei, the core functions of burials in facilitating a transition to the afterlife were never in doubt. They were just repackaged in a more consumerist and upbeat version of the ritual. State and police interventions at funerals after Covid offended communities not just because they took away families' rights to mourn or celebrate the lives of loved ones, but also because the rules and regulations prevented funerals from performing their core social functions: smooth passage to the afterlife with ritual care and social endorsement. It is difficult to comprehend the shock and horror that accompanied the imposition of the Covid regulations at funerals in the rural Eastern Cape between April and August 2020. The discussion below provides a sense of this experience.

Before Covid, it was considered undesirable to have more than one burial per day. Rural funerals were generally large affairs, attracting crowds of several hundred people, including kin, neighbours and urban visitors. In the week before the funeral weekend, young women from the village helped the family prepare the homestead and food for the guests while young men dug the grave. After the body arrived from the city or was fetched (*ukulanda umzimba*) from the local mortuary, it would normally be washed by young women. The ritual (*ukukhululwa kwezikhwenkwane*) was performed while the elders and family members delivered messages to the deceased to prepare them for safe passage to the afterlife. The body would have been dressed in "new clothes" (*ukunxibisa*) in preparation for display during the funeral rites. This sometimes took place at the local mortuary, where the body was dressed by selected family members. If the person was a church member, they would be dressed in their church uniform.

The night before the funeral, the body would be placed in the main house in the homestead where members of the immediate family and sometimes close friends would communicate with the deceased and prepare the spirit for its passage. They would recall their life and achievements in private; religious leaders might also join the vigil. The formal funeral would start early the next morning as the body was moved to a tent in the yard where a larger gathering would assemble. The coffin would normally be closed to avoid exposing the deceased to a wider public, some of whom, harbouring feelings of jealousy and envy, might want to bewitch the body. Trusted close friends and family would share their last thoughts and respects in the house, before the wider public arrived. A funeral programme might have included as many as a dozen speakers, including family, friends, neighbours, colleagues, religious leaders and a speaker from the house of traditional leaders. The actual funeral would have taken many hours as each person on the programme had their say. Many would affirm that the deceased caused no ill or harm to the community while alive. Thereafter, the religious leaders would walk with the coffin to the grave site as they spoke of the life after death. As the body was lowered into the grave, handfuls of soil were tossed into the grave, a practice known as *ukuthela umhlaba*, to symbolise the passage from dust to dust. Thereafter the guests would gather back in the tent and in the yard of the homestead where they would be fed and offered traditional beer and other beverages. This process could continue for the entire afternoon and evening after the burial in the morning.

Closing the gate: When custom causes Covid

The lockdown rules stated that funerals were not allowed to have more than 50 guests, that they had to be sanitised and social distanced, that a register of all attendees should be kept, that funerals should be reported to the police and that the funeral service could not take more than two hours. The body of the deceased could not be accessible to the family or mourners because any form of contact with the body was assumed to spread infection. Alcohol could also not be served because the customary practices of passing beakers of beer around at funerals was deemed extremely dangerous. These measures were extended to include the wrapping of bodies in plastic and even sealing the coffin itself in plastic to add further protection. The customary night vigils that occurred on the evening before the funeral and often went on through the night were also outlawed to stop families from opening the coffin, washing the body and trying to communicate with the deceased to assist them in their passage to the afterlife. On the day of the funeral, coffins were to be delivered, usually to the burial site instead of the tent or the house. Funeral parlour workers were dressed in hazmat suits and often brought canisters of sanitiser before the funeral to spay the premises. In some instances, they would arrive at the house just as the funeral guests arrived. The visual impact of men in white suits moving around the yard with spray guns was confusing and intimidating, especially since none of this was clearly explained to rural communities, who had all sorts of theories about where Covid came from and what it could do. This cluster of regulations and even the explanation of what the Covid-19 pandemic was were not widely shared with local communities, especially not in local languages or through local leaders and authorities. Many traditional leaders were reluctant to hold meetings and share the new government rules because they knew they would be unpopular. Some of the most common statements from the traditional leaders in these communities were as follows:

> we were not consulted by the government to represent our people's views and in knowing what is to be done so we can explain to the people, but we were reduced in the eyes of the people as we were not able to respond to their questions and issues, simply because we had no information to share to answer or calm their fears; in some instances during funeral gatherings, Covid virus is [seen to be] caused by our customs, because the state is at war with us and our customs. We were chased by the police, together with the people who are supposed to govern us, and we had to run in confusion; the way these regulations are expressed and the law enforcement that accompanies them against funerals and customs is as if this was all caused by us.

As a result, secrecy, fear and rumour dominated the rural landscape. People soon tired of coming to terms with the pandemic at the local level, since little information was provided in a format that would allow them to appreciate why some of the rules were imposed. They were consequently taken by complete surprise in April when the police arrived in numbers at funerals to enforce the Covid regulations.

In April 2020, community representatives across the former Transkei reflected on cases where the police had interfered in family funeral and customary rituals. They were extremely critical of what they considered to be a repressive campaign of intimidation by the state. One traditional leader recalled a case that was brought to his attention, where the family faced the dilemma of either obeying the rules of the state, or honouring the wishes of the deceased family patriarch:

During the beginning of the lockdown, people were afraid of the police and the military army. There was a household where the grandfather died, and while he was still alive, he said to the kids that during his funeral they should slaughter a cow and eight sheep. And they [the children] did exactly that to pay respect to their father's wishes. Many people went to that funeral, but the police came and chased them away. They said that only 50 members should attend. I believe that those family members knew about the rules, but they felt that spiritual consequences of not obeying their father was greater than not obeying the police. It is our culture that people are always afraid of not respecting the wish of the dead people. They consider that as caused bad luck and misfortune in the family.[40]

Social media coverage also indicated significant conflict between local people and police at funerals. At one funeral in Engcobo, police were reported to have acted violently, turning over pots that contained cooked food, meat and "*umqombothi*", the African home-made beer which is brewed as part of the funeral rituals. They also chased away mourners to keep the numbers down. Later on the same day, a police car carrying officers from the Engcobo funeral overturned on the road—which was interpreted as an act of vengeance by the ancestors, punishing the police for failing to respect the precepts of their own African culture at the funeral earlier.

In another complaint against the police, one respondent from the Kentani area claimed that the "local authorities and police would not allow the body, which had arrived from Cape Town, to enter the main house or the funeral tent". They reported that the authorities insisted that the body remained outdoors and was put in the ground as soon as possible. This caused great consternation for the family and relatives, who proclaimed that the deceased could not pass on to the next world under such stressful conditions and without communicating with the immediate family.

The clampdown by the police in the rural Transkei was part of a national campaign, sending out a message from the government that the lockdown measures were not optional. One traditional leader from the same area explained that: "there was a funeral at a neighbour's house, where more than 100 people gathered". The authorities took exception and raided the venue while the traditional healer was still in communication with the deceased. He explained: *ndithe ndisathetha uba lomfana lo ndiyamazi, kwathwa nanga amapolisa ndathi Haiboooo, sabaleka sonke*—"I was still talking about the deceased and someone shouted police! Police! And the law enforcement officials entered, and we all ran away".[41] The traditional leader said that the unannounced raid by the police undermined the process of communicating with the deceased and thus threatened the legitimacy of the funeral.

The police wanted rural communities to realise that the regulations were compulsory, and they seemed intent on instilling a climate of fear. The message was that those who did not obey the new rules would soon find themselves in jail; this will be further explored in chapter six.

Over the Easter weekend in 2020, many were offended by the way police behaved in rural areas, chasing people away from ceremonies and turning over drums of home-brewed beer. Rural communities felt they had not been consulted and that there had been no public education about the nature and risk of Covid-19. There had also been little communication among national, provincial and local officials on how to manage communities in rural areas. As lockdown enveloped rural communities, many felt as though they were caught in a tower of Babel—surrounded by the noise of new regulations and required changes in behaviours, but with little credible information and advice. The police were following their instructions to enforce the regulations and disperse large social gatherings; while the traditional leadership in the province independently announced that male initiation and customary ceremonies would be suspended until further notice. All funerals had to be reported to the police, who were required to be present at the funeral to ensure that rules and regulations were enforced. Chaos and confusion ensued as families and mourners had to confront the regulations, which made little sense to them and their understanding of custom. At numerous funerals attended by our co-researchers, local people said that the police and government were intervening to "mess up" the rituals, so that the spirits of the deceased would become confused and wander off course. The police commander in Engcobo acknowledged people's feelings that the police were "destroying their traditions" and had been sent to do this by the government. Communities wondered why traditional leaders were not coming out to support their people. One man explained: "we had many years of struggling with the AIDS, but when somebody died of AIDS, they were buried in the same way as anyone else". He concluded: "it is not like this Coronavirus because HIV never change our traditions, yes people were scared of AIDS, but at least they could be buried with dignity".[42]

Almost as if to justify the actions taken, at the end of April it was reported that 40 people had tested positive for Covid-19 in the village of Machibini in the Port St. Johns area of the former Transkei.[43] The state claimed the Machibini cases could be directly traced back to a funeral that had taken place in the village of Majola on 21 March, before the national lockdown started. This funeral, along with two others in the city of Port Elizabeth, were said to have accounted for 200 Covid-19 cases in the Eastern Cape—about a quarter of the provincial total at the time.[44] The media narrative around the outbreak in Port St. Johns pointed the finger at rural residents, who were portrayed as irredeemably selfish: "villagers—including some of those who are infected—do not seem to care", reported the region's *Daily Dispatch* newspaper. "The chaotic situation in Machibini village, where there is virtually no policing or army boots on the ground, is threatening to realise the health authorities' worst nightmare about a virus explosion in the province's rural areas".[45] In response to these concerns, King Zwelozuko Matiwane suspended all gatherings in villages of the AmaMpondomise Kingdom, including funerals and night vigils.[46] Clarifying the decision, the AmaMpondomise spokesperson, Nkosi Bakhanyisele Ranuga did reinstate the old tradition of *ukuqhusheka* in which the body was taken straight to the graveyard, although the body could be accompanied by no more than ten family members.

As the Covid-19 crisis intensified in the Eastern Cape, the government restrictions on funerals tightened even further. The period between death and burial was shortened and new cuts to the number of mourners were introduced. There were also further measures insisting that all bodies were tested for Covid-19, despite WHO advice that Covid bodies were not infectious after death.[47] The most controversial new measures that the funeral parlours enforced— partly for the safety of their own workers—were the placement of dead bodies in triple body bags to avoid contagion, and the prevention of families from viewing bodies before burial. This created further anxiety and confusion in rural areas. Some older men and women could not recall a time when the state had wanted to dictate how families performed their customs. They felt that the state regulations made it extremely difficult to bury the dead in culturally appropriate ways and to ensure safe passage for their loved ones to the afterlife.

Case studies collected in communities in the former Transkei reveal that restricted access to viewing and interaction with the corpse were a major source of anxiety. The regulations stipulated that the bodies of Covid-19 victims should not be accessible at funerals, especially not inside the house. Even when buried in a coffin, the bodies were supposed to be wrapped in solid plastic. In June 2020 a large funeral took place in the Kwa-Nikhwe village in Bizana. The body only arrived on the morning of the funeral, and the funeral service and rituals took place in the tent without the body present. When it arrived the body was taken straight to the gravesite, where it was buried before the funeral guests could bid their final farewells.[48] This incident elicited considerable complaints from attendees, but the funeral parlour said it would have lost its licence if it had broken the law. Multiple similar incidents occurred, including at Maya Location in Qamata, Chris Hani district. The passengers of two Quantum taxis from Cape Town arrived at the funeral to see the body but were told that the funeral parlour had taken the body straight to the gravesite.[49] In another case from the Mbashe municipality in a location near Willowvale town, the shortened funeral service and burial were completed before senior family members arrived from Johannesburg. The family was extremely angry because they had travelled a great distance to bid farewell and were unable to communicate with the deceased before their passage to the afterlife.[50] In at least one instance recorded in the Sinqumeni location in Engcobo, families became so angry at the way their burial rites were compromised by restrictions that they secretly exhumed the bodies after the police and mourners had left. They then reburied the body after removing the protecting plastic and communicating with the deceased.

During lockdown, when alcohol was prohibited, local police raided several funerals to overturn drums of *mqomboti* (traditional beer). The sharing of beer and food is critical to the communal ethos of *ubuntu* at funerals. Beer is also needed to reward the gravediggers, whose spades and picks are symbolically washed in "soothing" traditional beer. In other cases, authorities attempted to shorten funerals to prevent people from lingering. In June, at a funeral at Bhongweni village in Tsolo in the uMhlontlo municipality, the body arrived from Johannesburg at 4 am. In the dark, the family welcomed neighbours to view the body. The next day, 50 people attended the funeral as stipulated under the Covid-19 restrictions. Fearing prosecution, they shortened the funeral to under two hours, and according to the mother only two people had spoken. Later, she spoke of regretting the decision because the funeral had felt "incomplete".[51] In Kentani, meanwhile, an old woman died in her 90s after serving as a prominent community leader. She was much loved and respected. At the time of her death in July 2020, the entire village community were ready and eager to attend the funeral to show their respects. The problem was that only 50 people could be invited to attend the ceremony, and only one or two representatives were able to speak at the funeral, which left much unsaid and many behind the homestead gate. The person who shared this story recalled that on the day of the funerals there were over a hundred people gathered in the street outside. They had come to listen and participate as best they could "from afar".

In a setting where the size of local funerals had previously grown, keeping numbers down to 50 meant that many people who should have attended were left uninvited. Vuyokazi from Willowvale explained that the whole question of invitation was confusing because funerals were traditionally open events, meaning that anyone in the village could attend if they wished to show their respects. They were always popular because foods and beverages were always available. In most of the locations in the former Transkei, local headmen were careful to allow only one funeral per weekend so as not to split the loyalty of locals to different families. They did not want people to have to miss paying their respects at one funeral because they were committed to attending another. As the pandemic took hold in the Eastern Cape during the middle of 2020, and especially during the second wave over December 2020 and January 2021, it was no longer possible for this rule to be maintained. As a result, funerals were held throughout the week, and sometimes almost every day, to manage the number of burials needed. One woman from Lusikisiki explained in an interview in December 2020: "there are now more death than days of week in this location. I am not sure what the headmen will do now".

The state's decision to limit the number of mourners was by far the most contentious issue. In all ten municipalities where fieldwork was undertaken, families complained bitterly about this ruling. Some understood the need for reducing the numbers at funerals but said that it was insensitive to apply a single rule to all cases because the people who died were of different ages and standing in the community. They did not believe the state or police had a right to determine who could attend a funeral, insiting that this was essentially a family or at least local community decision. They felt that older, more senior members of the community—who had returned from the cities long ago and and were very well known and respected—deserved more recognition than a young man who had not yet contributed much to the home. Some police intervention in these areas occured when families reported that they would only have 50 at the funeral but did not turn mourners away on the day, allowing dozens more than the prescribed number to gather. The police would then arrive and ask all those who were not on the list to leave. When they resisted the police often took harsh action, driving people away by force or overturning food and beer pots. The other issue that confused mourners was the requirement that they wash their hands on entering the yard. Traditionally, hands were only washed at the grave site, when mourners would wash their hands in a mixture of water and the bile of an ox (*inyongo*) as a concluding gesture. This was also known as "washing the spades" and was associated with drinking beer in recognition of the communal labour of the young men who dug the grave. The idea that hands needed to be repeatedly washed at the beginning and during the service seemed peculiar to many, as it implied the ritual was coming to an end even before it had started.

The other issue that concerned mourners was the confusion surrounding the arrival of the body in the morning. They expected the body to have been collected from the mortuary the day before, and blessed, washed and clothed while close relatives, friends and spiritual leaders spoke to the deceased and put them at ease. The ritual service, which usually began at 10 pm, was known as *unlindelo* or *inkonzo yokuqala*. It gave the family a chance to say their final goodbyes in an intimate setting. In the absence of this process, mourners still expected some welcoming of the body when it arrived at the homestead. They mentioned a practice called *ulwamkela umzimba*, wherein family members would do a short prayer and welcome the deceased home before proceeding to the tent or the grave site. The fact that the funeral parlours were only delivering the deceased on the same day, often while the acknowledgments were being made in the tent or the yard, proceeding straight to the grave site and burying the body before the mourners could arrive was regarded as appalling. It essentially meant that the deceased went into the ground without being welcomed home. The transit of the spirit from the city or local mortuary was a delicate affair, as explained above. There was always the chance that the spirit could be confused along the way and wander, like a lost ghost, into the wilderness. The spirit needed to be nurtured, welcomed home and constantly reassured that their life had been worthy, and that they were recognised and respected, so that they could then move onto the afterlife with ease. The Covid rules were not adapted to meet these expectations, or even communicated clearly to communities in rural areas.[52]

In the preparations for a funeral, feeding the guests was a complex cultural process which involved planning and ensuring that the best cuts from the sacrificial beast were distributed amongst the most senior men and close kin, who were also served first. Careful consideration of seniority and gender was observed in matters involving the distribution of food and beer. The consumption and spilling of homebrewed beer at the homestead was always an invitation to the ancestors to visit, which was especially needed at times of death. The seating arrangements at the funeral also reflected status and hierarchy, based on an acknowledgement of gender and generational divisions. Senior women would direct proceedings in the preparation of food and making of traditional beer. This would start days before the actual funeral. The young women or *makotis* (young brides) would usually wash and dress the body during the night vigil, as well as work diligently on the preparation of food. On the day of the funeral, they would also be expected to serve the guests, placing themselves, as Sharpley argues, at the frontline of possible infection.[53] Young men would be responsible for digging the grave and assisting with the slaughtering of the sacrificial beast, which usually occurred on the Thursday before the funeral at the weekend.[54] With the banning of alcohol and the restriction of the number of attendees, the critical social process of collective consumption at the funeral was terminated as families now prepared food parcels for guests to take home with them once the funeral service was complete and the body buried. Additional packages were prepared for mourners who came to the gate or sat against the fence outside the yard.[55]

The absence of senior chiefs and traditional leaders at the funeral also frequently occurred during the first wave of Covid in the Eastern Cape.[56] As mentioned above, traditional leaders were civil servants and therefore instructed to enforce the Covid rules and regulations. In the Eastern Cape, both the regional House of Traditional Leaders and the Congress of Traditional Leaders of South Africa publicly endorsed the Covid rules and regulations, confirming that customary practices would cease in their territorials and that funerals would comply with the Covid rules. But when they realised how opposed people were to the regulations, and how much trauma they were causing in local communities, senior traditional leaders stayed away from funerals and out of the public eye. Many of our respondents felt that in the context of all the changes, local people were looking to senior traditional leaders to give them assurance. They did not want to see a young, junior chief or local headman standing in for the senior traditional leader in the area. Some people believed the traditional leaders stayed away because they feared infection, and sent younger men who would stand more chance of surviving Covid. Village residents were also highly critical of urban elites in the ruling African National Conference (ANC), who seemed to have forgotten about the rural poor. These elites hosted funerals in the cities that did not conform to the attendance limits that were so strictly imposed in the rural areas. Rural elites, like traditional leaders, had limits placed on their funerals that were not imposed at the funerals of political elites in the city, which generated much discussion and controversy. Rural communities expected elites and very elderly senior people to get concessions, much as the ANC elites did in the cities.

By the end of June 2020, the wrapping of bodies in three layers of plastic and the delivery of bodies directly to graves had become common practice, creating enormous anxiety in rural areas. In the Zixhoseni location, one woman explained that: "as Xhosa people, we bury our family members in a way that they can come and visit us after death at our homes, and to do this they need to be free, not wrapped in plastic".[57] Another mourner said that: "I can say that our normal way of doing things are disturbed by these Covid rules, because during funerals it is not our culture to wrap people in plastic".[58] The local community leaders added that: "I can say that it is affecting people emotionally because family expect to be able to communicate with the body at the home, and in other ways before they are buried, but this is not possible through plastic".[59] Another mourner said that wrapping bodies in plastic caused the spirit of the dead person to become "overheated", creating misfortune and chaos.[60] One ward councillor pointed out that the triple plastic covering made it difficult for people to determine who was in the bag, and that this had led to the wrong corpse being buried in multiple cases. He quoted a well-known incident where the wrong body had been sent from Cape Town to Cofimvaba for burial, while the Cofimvaba body ended up in KwaZulu-Natal.[61] Local residents said that these errors were made because so many nurses, doctors and government bureaucrats were on strike and there were "no longer qualified people to register the dead".[62] In a number of instances, communities chased the funeral parlour vehicle away from the homestead because of the alien and unacceptable state in which the body was delivered, wrapped in plastic.

Conclusion

The police crackdown at funerals which was strictly enforced across rural areas in April and May 2020 started to taper off in June and July, when rural infections peaked. As time passed, some families did manage to negotiate specific arrangements with the local authorities and police for more guests to attend or for a longer funeral service to be held. The crackdown in April was clearly intended as shock therapy. As a result, the intensity naturally tapered off, and we recorded many cases where some special concession or arrangement was made with the authorities to allow the service to be extended to make space for more eulogies, or the numbers attending to be increased by 20 or 30. But as the death rate increased rapidly in May, June and July the face of bio-medicine and the state shifted from the police to the funeral parlours. They were required to enforce extremely unpopular regulations, like the delivery of the body on the same day as the funeral, the burial of bodies before the mourners could reach the grave side and the frightening rituals of sanitising house and grave sites. In April 2020, we were told by a police chief in Engcobo that the people felt the police were deliberately "messing up" their rituals and disturbing the ancestors. The palpable anger of local communities was seen in numerous acts of defiance which provoked even more coercive action, as images circulated like wildfire on social media. By June and July, the focus on popular anger had shifted from the police to funeral parlours, now seen as the frontline of the state's attempt to implement such insensitive and damaging regulations. Some funeral parlours seemed to have decided to bury bodies without mourners present to avoid engaging the wrath of the communities, who started chasing funeral parlour vans and were threatening to assault their personnel.[63]

The argument of this chapter is that the first round of state and bio-medical intervention in South Africa was extremely traumatic for rural communities. Not only did they find that local health facilities were shutting down around them as the infection rates increased, as the next chapter will explore, but they experienced a great deal of anxiety around the state's interventions and regulations around their funerals and customary practices. Indeed, during the first wave of Covid-19 infection in the Eastern Cape, we argued that lockdown bought high levels of fear, panic and marginalisation in rural communities. They felt that the state was "closing the gate on them", both literally and figuratively. The chapter has focused on rural funeral practices and illustrated how significant rural home burial remains in a context of rapid social change in the society. Families who originate from the rural areas of the Eastern Cape still predominantly wish to bring the bodies of their loved ones home for burial in a family and community ceremony at the rural homestead. These ceremonies could be large and extravagant, depending on the wealth of the family and the extent of their funeral cover and life insurance. During Covid, there was a great deal of confusion around rural funerals, which were restricted to 50 participants and controlled by the rules of the state and funeral parlours. Rural families were not used to being told how to run their family rituals. They wondered whether their kin would ever find peace in regulated events where rites of passage could not be observed as expected and bodies were sealed in plastic bags. At a workshop held in November 2020, a representative from the Eastern Cape House of Traditional Leaders said that the House was inundated with cases of families wanting to rebury family members. They felt that they could no longer cope with the way the Covid restrictions had disrupted their genealogies of connection to place, and the dignity of their families and communities. As one man explained: "people are not dead until they have a funeral; it is only them that we know who they really were and how to recover from their death".

3

DISPOSABLE CITIZENS

The bio-medical fix

After lockdown was declared in South Africa in March 2020, an early priority for the government in the Eastern Cape was to crack down on customary practices in rural areas, especially the former Ciskei and Transkei. The Eastern Cape House of Traditional Leaders supported the government's declaration of a state of disaster, the ban on customary practices and the new restrictions on funerals. At the end of March, the Eastern Cape House of Traditional Leaders chair, Nkosi Mwelo Nonkonyana, urged traditional leaders and their rural subjects to take Covid-19 seriously. He stressed the potential danger and devastation that the Coronavirus could cause in rural communities if people failed to comply with the rules, especially to the elderly and the sick. At this time, the Contralesa provincial secretary, Nkosi Mkhanyiseli Dudumayo, also stated his concern that, while there was general observance of the lockdown rules in urban areas, in rural areas people were going about their lives as normal. The message seemed to be that defiant rural communities were unprepared to follow government rules. With the support of traditional leaders, and through the police force, the regional government embarked on a concerted effort from late March to May 2020 to crack down on rural communities and families who appeared to ignore the state's lockdown regulations. The lockdown situation was compounded in July 2020 as cases rose in rural areas. The provincial Premier Oscar Mabuyane intervened to tighten the regulations in the province, insisting that funeral services be limited to one hour only, that hospitals produce evidence of the cause of death and that funeral parlours take coffins directly to the grave sites in rural areas.

Academic and policy analyst Steven Friedman was astonished at the path the government had become entrapped on. The decision to tighten population controls and imitate Northern bio-medical scientific approaches could not be replicated in South Africa outside of a few metropolitan centres, which had the capacity for hi-tech tracking, testing, and tracing.[1] Friedman argued that the ruling and urban middle classes admired Western consumerist lifestyles and seemed determined to follow the Northern bio-medical model, instead of acknowledging the limitations of the country's science and public health infrastructure. Some other governments in the global South and Africa had tried to forge their own response based on an assessment of their resources, capacities and situations.[2] But the ruling African National Congress (ANC), supported by the corporate private sector, seemed determined to align with the hi-tech and bio-medical approaches of the global North. Friedman also claimed that the ruling party knew they would not be able to keep pace with the North, but wanted to keep the belief alive. They thus tightened controls over the local population so that the virus would not spread to expose the weakness in the system.[3] He argued that the ANC government knew that it was involved in sleight of hand that would be difficult to maintain. The President, the Minister of Health and their advisory council of top doctors and scientists focused on hospitals, and finding private sector support for new field hospitals to absorb the expected surge of treatment needed in the cities. The rural healthcare system, in contrast, was ignored and barely mentioned in the media throughout the first wave.

This out-of-reach, top-down, bio-medical fix, driven by an advisory council comprised only of medical doctors and scientists, had catastrophic effects in the rural periphery. One crisis catalysed the next, leading to a chain of events that shut down government and the health care system. In July 2021, a years after the first wave, Estelle Ellis—a senior journalist at the *Daily Maverick* and award-winning expert on

Covid in South Africa—reported the provincial Covid mortality rates were amongst the highest in the world. She wrote that:

> according to the (Health) department's own epidemiological records, Buffalo City metro has the highest mortality rate at 293.6/100,000, followed by the Nelson Mandela metro at 273.5/100,000 and the Chris Hani (rural) district at 209.1/100,000. Compared with the World Health Organization's Covid-19 data, these rates are among the highest in the world and significantly higher than those of Italy (175/100,000), the US (166/100,000), Spain (157/100,000) and Brazil (142/100,000).[4]

This chapter will explain how tunnel vision, oversight and arrogance produced these death rates. Covid had a devastating impact in the province, both in the two main metropolitan areas, Nelson Mandela Bay and Buffalo City, and across the rural landscape, with rates in excess of 200 deaths per 100,000 people. This chapter argues that these death rates were a product of the social dynamics of the region's migrant labour system and the spectacular failure of the state's public health approach, which escalated the problem through a series of knock-on effects that left people and institutions unprotected. The chapter documents the unfolding crisis during the first wave of infection in South Africa. Between April and August 2020, hospital and clinic staff shortages, fear, poor preparation, lack of equipment and the absence of community engagement brought the urban and rural health systems to a standstill. Many government departments, including those that issued the death certificates required for funeral insurance, were closed. The chapter explores how medical mayhem deepened fear and uncertainty in rural communities, and how the specific medical regime that was implemented failed to protect or care for the rural poor. It illustrates how the shift from a bare life to a naked life can be achieved through neglect as well as intent. To return to the theories of Agamben, the case material presented here shows quite clearly that under regimes of exception the state is prepared to sacrifice souls, disposing of lives and bodies, to allow those in power to maintain their regime of privilege and control. One journalist invoked the image of Dante's inferno, where the damned were left to burn.[5]

In explaining how different factors intersected, the chapter explores how confusion and alienation spread in the rural areas. It also illustrates how families and communities ultimately developed their own coping strategies to counteract the strategies of the state, including the use of indigenous knowledge, community networks and traditional healers, who had been shut out of the state's bio-medical regime for the management of Covid-19. The chapter does acknowledge the efforts of the state to provide social support for the poor through a national R100 billion relief package announced in July 2020. However, these grants were only administered through post offices in towns, many of which did not operate efficiently in the rural areas and were affected by the general shutdown of government services.[6] The struggles to access these grants are well documented in the media and reveal that no special effort was made to ensure that the rural poor had the same access as those in urban areas, who could also access the internet for applications. The exclusion of rural people from access to opportunities was a product of both the long-term structural violence of colonialism, as Farmer would call it, and also the short-term expediency of an imported bio-medical model that was disconnected from local realities.[7]

Colonial hospitals, nurses and rural healthcare

In the late 19th century, the rural healthcare infrastructure in the Eastern Cape seemed to punch above its weight. Numerous small mission hospitals and clinics were constructed in the eastern half of the region as the frontier was consolidated as part of the "civilising mission" of European Christianity and British colonialism. Rural hospitals stressed better care for rural Africans and sought to modernise rural hygiene, while also containing disease and reforming local belief systems. The missionary influence in the Eastern Cape ensured that outstanding institutions, like Victoria Hospital in Alice and Holy Cross Mission and Hospital in Flagstaff, emerged as regional anchors, setting the tone for rural healthcare in colonial Africa in the early 20th century.[8] The Victoria Hospital in Alice also prioritised the training of professional African nurses, emerging as a sister institution next to the University of Fort Hare. Eminent South African historian Shula Marks argued that, by the end of the 19th century, nursing in South Africa was dominated primarily by English women who migrated to the country to fulfil the higher demands of health care brought about by industrial change.[9] With them, they brought the image of the "lady nurse", which embedded ideas about caring as intrinsically linked with femininity and moral duty: "not only would the sisterhood provide nursing care; their purity and devotion would provide the necessary moral example".[10]

In the rural African context, nursing services were provided predominantly by religious sisterhoods and were accompanied by a particular ethos modelled on Victorian notions of femininity and Christian duty. The anthropologist Elizabeth Hull stresses how propaganda from the colonial government reinforced the idea of the "nurturing female role", a quintessential aspect of nursing. The government's insistence on the God-given duty of all women to provide care was part of a broader colonial strategy of managing labour resources. In the early 20th century, mission-educated nursing provided one of the few avenues for upward mobility and elite social status for women.[11] For the colonial government, nurses represented a desired transition to Western forms of medicine and healthcare, which were deeply embedded within a broader moral and ideological project of "civilizing the natives". This project depended on the eradication of "superstitious" and "ignorant" traditional beliefs. Therefore, Marks suggests, the black nurses at this time constituted the ideal colonial subject. They represented "harbingers of progress and healing in black society, a shining light in the midst of its savagery and disease".[12]

In the Eastern Cape, there was no more prestigious calling for African women in colonial society than nursing. The province was renowned nationally for the high quality of its nursing staff and training institutions, like Victoria Hospital in Alice and Frere Hospital in East London. Many of the mission-trained nurses from this generation also became the wives of the African-educated elites who took leadership roles in the ANC and the liberation movement. The social bonds among the nurses played a critical role in forging a common sense of identity and purpose among this generation of leaders. In this sense, the colonial healthcare system was at the forefront of notions of African modernity and development. The beautiful and professionally turned-out nurses epitomised the image of a new class of African civil servants who would lead the continent to independence, lifting

African people to a new state of modernity. However, as Marks notes, there was a fundamental contradiction for nurses between the values they were expected to project in their professional life and their position as African women in a patriarchal, racially divided colonial society.[13] In her work on Holy Cross Hospital, Diana Wylie shows how official attitudes to Africans' hunger hardened with the arrival of apartheid, changing from a paternalist "*noblesse oblige*" to a less sympathetic "they must not be spoiled" stance.[14] The treatment of Africans as units of labour meant that the definition of hunger was under constant revision, as South Africa moved toward apartheid-style "high modernism" underpinned by scientific racism.[15]

In South Africa today, nursing as a profession no longer enjoys the same status and prestige, and does not offer guarantees of rapid upward social mobility into the middle class. In her book *Contingent Citizens*, Elizabeth Hull explores the shift from missionary, faith-based and caring institutions based on Eurocentric and Victorian traditions, which dominated the first half of the 20th century, to the secularisation of nursing and its ethos from the introduction of apartheid to the present. While the apartheid state shut down mission schools in the 1950s and replaced them with state schools and Bantu Education, it did not do the same to mission hospitals. There were no trained black doctors to replace the white ones, so a hybrid system emerged in which rural health care was caught between the state and the church.[16] The state continued to use the mission system, but no longer offered financial support. Consequently, rural hospitals were run in confusing ways. They remained *de facto* mission-led institutions, but operated under boards and systems established by the apartheid state and homeland authorities, which controlled funding. A process of decentralisation and secularisation accelerated during the 1970s and 1980s, as rural health care was expanded through a network of clinics in the countryside. The focus was on expanding access to basic healthcare. The movement of nurses out of the hospital environment and its network of clinics increased state control and downgraded the status of nurses; they became lower-level state functionaries instead of high-prestige professionals. In the context of this change, Hull notes that many of the older nurses she interviewed were nostalgic about the "old days", when African nurses were high-status workers and valued members of the African middle class.[17]

During the post-apartheid period, the state expanded the focus on primary healthcare provision in rural areas through the Reconstruction and Development Programme (RDP) and the consolidation of basic services at rural clinics. A countrywide drive aimed to expand the infrastructure of rural clinics and better manage rural health with new systems of monitoring and evaluation. In the 1990s, the rural health care system came under severe strain with the outbreak of the HIV and AIDS pandemic and the tuberculosis crisis in this migrant-sending area. Nurses now felt undervalued and over-worked across the system. Hull argues that the state simply treated them as units of labour to be managed within a large, unrewarding bureaucratic system. Nurses themselves began to widely recognise that standards were dropping, and their professionalism was being increasingly compromised by the HIV and AIDS pandemic and massification. They also felt that the state had failed to attend to professional training, nursing hierarchies and advancement.[18]

From the time of democracy, the public health system in the new Eastern Cape province came under intense pressure from the subcontinental spread of the HIV and AIDs pandemic. The power of the deeply entrenched circular migration system drove infections, while low levels of urban permanence, which persisted into democracy, meant that many of the chronically sick left the cities and returned to the rural areas when they became seriously ill. This posed an enormous burden on rural households and communities, especially since people with HIV and AIDS were also stigmatised in the rural areas. Paul Farmer has written about the role of the structural violence of slavery, colonial and resource extraction in West Africa and the burden it has placed on the rural poor. The migrant labour system produced a similar legacy in southern Africa, as rural families were broken up by long periods of separation and under-development. When the democratic government tried to extend the public health services in rural areas after apartheid, it was hamstrung by enormous challenges and pressure on the ground. As time passed, the ANC was increasing criticised for lack of community engagement, critical staff shortages, the poor quality of services at hospitals and clinics, departmental inefficiency, corruption and a lack of basic medicines, especially at rural clinics. While the provincial government promised new management systems, better infrastructure, and new staff across the system, the Eastern Cape Department of Health struggled on into the new millennium, surviving with support from external experts and funds from international donor groups.

One significant development in the 2000s was the relocation of the headquarters of the Treatment Action Campaign (TAC) from Cape Town to Lusikisiki in the Eastern Cape.[19] The TAC clashed with the Eastern Cape Department of Health over a number of issues, especially since they adopted a more activist and community-centred approach, which put the Department on the defensive.[20] The deteriorating relations between the provincial Department and NGOs and activist groups in the rural health sector ultimately resulted in the formation of the Eastern Cape Health Crisis Coalition (ECHCC) in 2013. The ECHCC produced a damning report on the state of public health in the province, entitled *Death and Dying in the Eastern Cape*. It detailed a litany of health rights violations that frequently resulted in death, including crumbling infrastructure, the lack of essential medication across the sector, critical supply chains weakness, the lack qualified staff and the poor management of hospitals.[21] In addition, the report found that issues like basic contract management for outsourced food and laundry were neglected, that new medical equipment was being procured to replace broken or old equipment, and that the department failed to appoint or pay clinical staff on time, causing critical understaffing.[22] In 2018, the TAC revisited the 2013 report of the ECHCC and found that nothing had improved in the five years since the report was submitted to the provincial department.

When the government committed itself to a first world bio-medical approach to the pandemic in 2020, it was immediately clear that the Eastern Cape Health Department would not be able to meet the technical and scientific management requirements. By early April 2020, the national Minister of Health, Zwide Mkhize, was already reprimanding the Eastern Cape Health Department for providing figures on tracing, testing and screening for Covid-19 that "simply did not add up".[23] At the end of April, the Minister and a full delegation from his national department visited the Nelson Mandela Bay, the main metropolitan areas in the province, to get a first-hand account. They found that there were only two qualified infectious disease experts in a province of 6 million people, more than 6,000 staff vacancies in the public health sector, including thousands of critical staff, and a lack of available Personal Protective Equipment (PPE), which made instituting safely measures and managing quarantine difficult. When Mkhize left the province, he remained optimistic that the bio-medical system could be rehabilitated in time for the first surge of infections. He promised 10 epidemiologists to help the provincial government manage the pandemic, as well as military doctors from the defence force to be put on standby to support the region. He argued that:

> I believe that the team that has now come from the national office is going to give us a coherent strategy on how to manage the infections, the outbreak from district to district, and *I believe we have been able to make an adequate intervention to unlock movement going forward and containment in this area* (namely, the Eastern Cape).[24]

In the next two months, he made numerous additional visits to the province and promised to shore up technical and management support for the main urban hospitals in the region, especially Livingston Hospital in Port Elizabeth and Cecilia Makiwane Hospital in East London. But the largest rate of infection rate in the province was not in the two metros, but in the rural interior where the two former homelands, the Ciskei and the Transkei, were located. It was mainly during the second wave, when the more infectious South African 'Beta' variant emerged during December 2020 and January 2021, that the high density urban populations and the December home-coming to the Eastern Cape accelerated rates of infection astronomically in the metros. Nelson Mandela Bay and Buffalo City were always high-profile infection zones, but little attention was ever focused on addressing the rural Covid challenge in the province and the country. In the discussion below, we briefly turn our attention to the crisis at Livingstone Hospital, and how it deteriorated rather than improved after the Minister's visit in April. We then shift our focus to the rural areas where there was effectively no public health system in operation during the first wave, or, as chapter six will detail, the second wave.

Livingstone Hospital: The eye of the storm

In her 2014 book, *Biomedicine in an Unstable Place,* Alice Street argues that public hospitals have long served as sites for imagining the state and, more broadly, modernity.[25] She claims that the collapse of a city, region or state's hospitals is always a critical indicator of the developmental capacity and resilience of the area. She argues that in Indonesia, especially in the country's more remote rural areas, the designation of regions as unstable, uncertain and under-developed is often simply "read" off the conditions at the local hospitals, which are generally deemed to be sub-standard, chaotic and disorderly in terms of the dominant Western bio-medical ideal of a modern hospital.[26] In the context of South Africa and the Covid pandemic, the Livingstone Hospital in the Eastern Cape city of Port Elizabeth became that place, defining the global view of the country and the management of the pandemic. It started in July 2020, when the hospital failed a safety inspection as the first wave of infection rates skyrocketed across the country and hospitals fell under scrutiny. Livingstone Hospital was already on the radar of journalists and the media because of Minister Mkize's visit to the facility in April, where he acknowledged provincial challenges but vowed to plug gaps by transferring specialist staff to the province.

In early July 2020, the *Daily Maverick* broke the story that the hospital had failed a safety inspection and that: "patients, visitors and employees at Port Elizabeth's Livingstone Hospital were met with the horrifying sight of rats licking at water the colour of blood pouring from a blocked drain" (see Figure 3).[27] Department of Health officials disputed the claim, saying that "an unknown person had put beetroot peels down the drain, causing the water to turn red".[28] The report found that sanitary condition of the hospital was appalling, with piles of rubbish and medical waste lining the passages, while patients slept wherever they could find space inside or outside the wards. The *Daily Maverick* claimed that the causality unit had warned in mid-June that conditions at the hospital were "dangerously unsanitary" and the none of the appointments promised when the Minister visited had been made.[29] Staff at the hospital had also embarked on a go-slow strike after a disagreement over overtime in June. The hospital was described as a rudderless, toxic and dangerous institution without proper protocols, PPE or protection from infection for staff or patients. Ntiski Mpulo from the ECHCC said that the conditions at Livingstone Hospital had "deteriorated catastrophically in recent times". The reports on Livingstone attracted the international media with a week-long visit from the BBC and reports on Sky News from the hospital and local cemeteries. Andrew Harding of the BBC found doctors and nurses at Livingstone Hospital to be exhausted and over-whelmed with Covid patients, some of whom were sleeping on newspapers on the floor. The hospital was out of oxygen and had a severe shortage of ambulances and ventilators; Harding described scenes from the hospital as "like a war zone".[30]

The BBC and Sky News beamed these images of the hospital in crisis across the globe in a series of special reports on the Covid-19 crisis in South Africa. The unwashed corridors and blood-stained wards with no staff revealed the extreme conditions prevalent in the Eastern Cape, the weakest link in a national healthcare system that was buckling under severe strain.[31] Livingstone Hospital came to represent the state of the province and the country. Dr Black, head of the infectious diseases unit at the hospital, reported that the institu-tion was down to 30% of its staff, and that there was a huge amount of fear and emotional and mental fatigue at the facility. He said that services were "starting to crumble under the strain" because "Covid-19 has opened up the cracks in the system—it has created a lot of conflict". Harding claimed that mothers and babies were dying in the nearby Dora Nginza Hospital, which had a large maternity ward. He quoted nurses saying that there were several mother and infant deaths every week, which had been unheard-of before Covid-19. Harding said that public sector unions had shut down hospital after hospital in the province and had refused to budge until their demands were met, leaving patients without care. While he felt that the public did not support the strike action, the nurses' unions and other professional bodies would not advise staff to return until conditions were safe. The piece ends by suggesting that the horror on display at the two hospi-tals was not a flash-in-the-pan but emblematic of a provincial health system and service which had been in a state of decline for the past 10 years. Harding viewed the hospital's poor conditions and dirty floors and linen as indicative of a larger national problem, as Alice Street would have predicted he might.

The failure of doctors and nurses at Livingstone Hospital to hold their ground in the face of the Covid-19 crisis provided a lasting image for the failure of Eastern Cape to manage the escalating pandemic, as it recorded more than 2,000 new infections a day by early July 2020. However, by using the hospital to represent the crisis in the province, the gaze of the media and the world was confined to conditions in the city, even though the vast majority of those living in the region were served by rural clinics. The threat presented to staff and patients by unsanitary conditions and the lack of PPE—represented at Livingstone by the image of rats licking blood at a drain—became the single most important issue that brought the healthcare system and the government to a standstill. Sterile environments were required in all government institutions.

Deep cleaning and the rural health crisis

The state's failure to "deep clean" infected public spaces came to the fore for the first time in the province in early May 2020, when Zwide clinic in Port Elizabeth closed down because one nurse had died and 11 others had tested positive for Covid-19.[32] The metro did not have the PPE equipment or staff willing to clean the facility properly, and only the pharmacy was deep cleaned. In response, the nurses complained to their union, who supported them in their refusal to return to an unsafe work environment. The Zwide clinic crisis proved to be the tip of the iceberg; public sector facilities closed like dominoes across the province because of reported infections. By mid-May, more than 10 police stations, mainly in the western part of the province, had been shuttered due to outbreaks and public safety concerns. Meanwhile, Home Affairs offices were also closed in the large metros and urban centres, together with several smaller rural hospitals and clinics in places such as Centane and Komga.[33]

Members of public sector unions, including the Police and Prisons Civil Rights Union (POPCRU), stood firm by refusing to return to work until their stations had been professionally, systematically cleaned. They refused to accept improper or partial cleaning. But in the absence of trained staff, appropriate equipment and professional systems to conduct proper deep cleaning, buildings could not be returned to functionality and many key parts of the health system and government were shut down. The closures were also partly a consequence of more rigorous testing for the virus among public servants, which revealed a significant number of cases. Notwithstanding the reasons for the shutdowns, public servants were criticised for not being available to assist those in need. People noted that the police were operating roadblocks without masks or protective gear and yet there seemed to be a general lack of commitment among public servants to re-open clinics, police stations and services to the public.

In the second half of May 2020, infections began to spike in the rural district municipalities of OR Tambo and Chris Hani. These areas had deep migration tracks in and out of Gauteng and Durban, in the case of OR Tambo, and Cape Town, Port Elizabeth and East London in the case of Chris Hani. This made them the first rural hotspots in South Africa and among the most vulnerable areas in the country. At this time, the situation at hospitals in East London and Mthatha was receiving increasing attention in the national media, especially in relation to their periodic closure and their shortages of PPE. Nurses claimed that these hospitals were still using the old green gowns, which were unsafe and should be replaced with appropriate PPE. Frere Hospital in East London and Mthatha Hospital both closed, as more and more people began to seek help.

By the end of July, the Eastern Cape had over 75,000 confirmed cases of Covid-19; more than 1,500 official Covid-19 deaths (and perhaps at least three times that amount unofficially); and 58,000 recoveries.[34] To compound matters, 3,500 health workers had tested positive for the virus and 56 had lost their lives. One Livingstone doctor summed it up as follows: "we have 1,200 beds for Covid-19 patients, but only 200 are oxygenated, and there are currently enough staff to serve 30 beds".[35] Another doctor stated that it was an impossible situation because: "You can't administer anything through them [the provincial health department] because it will go missing. It all boils down to the fact that the department is dysfunctional beyond belief and has no money."[36]

It was this recognition that led Mkhize to intervene again in mid-July. He aimed to create a new "turn-around strategy" with the support of his own adviser, Dr Sibongile Zungu—who was sent to join the Eastern Cape Covid-19 project management team—and the Eastern Cape Premier, Oscar Mabuyane. The premier supported the strategy with a new commitment of R2.5 billion from the provincial budget. He said that R840 million of this would go towards building field hospitals around the province; another R480 million would address backlogs in PPE; R173 million would fund the purchase of ventilators; R17 million would be spent on increasing the capacity of nursing staff; and R12 million would fund Cuban doctors brought into local hospitals to block the gaps.[37] It was also announced that 75 doctors from the National Defence Force would be relocated to the province.

Throughout this period, evidence of the poor conditions at rural hospitals increasingly came to light, especially in the media. In rural Centane, doctors and nurses were so deprived of drugs and PPE that they walked out of the hospital in early June, leaving patients in their beds. They told the media that they would no longer risk their lives daily because of the government's failure to implement PPE and the accepted standard operating procedures at their hospital. More than 100 people working at the hospital allegedly downed tools. They said that they would not return until they had access to PPE and the facility was disinfected, noting that one hospital clerk had already died and several other staff members were now critically ill. At the Frontier Provincial Hospital in Komani, nurses also went on strike because of the absence of PPE and their inability to control mentally ill patients, transferred from a nearby psychiatric hospital, who wandered the corridors and refused to follow rules. The action was taken after 56 nurses at the hospital had tested positive for Covid-19. It was supported by the Democratic Nurses Organisation of South Africa (DENOSA), which called for hospital's CEO to resign for allowing the facility to be overrun by Covid-19. These developments provoked rural nurses in clinics to follow suit and shut facilities until they were cleaned and staff could be tested.[38]

At Komga Hospital, families complained that their relatives had been left to care for themselves after the nurses there also walked out. The hospital was also allegedly no longer processing the paperwork required to release the bodies of patients who had died; relatives of the deceased, including the family of Anele Mxhosana, petitioned the health department to produce the appropriate paperwork.[39] The closure of hospitals and clinics created panic and anger in rural areas, and rural villagers were bitterly disappointed at the inability of the formal health system to address their needs. Many said that they had relied on traditional healers and local herbal remedies when they were unable to source help at their local clinics and hospitals. In other reports received from districts in the former Transkei, rural families complained about the failure of nurses to be ready or sympathetic, saying they lacked the capacity to provide essential services when rural "people needed them most". Statements like the following were common: "The nurses here only seem to care for themselves. You will not see them at the clinics. They are hiding away. The clinics are closed because they are scared." Others felt that the clinics did not have any dedicated information or strategy to deal with Covid-19; instead, they just referred people to the urban hospitals, which they could see were failing. Local people from prominent families were apparently talking about driving the sick to Durban, Cape Town or Johannesburg because of the lack of services available in the province. There is no doubt some truth to the statements that some nurses were not at their stations in rural clinics because of fear and uncertainty about the pandemic, and their perceived vulnerability to infection. However, closer investigation reveals that the criticism of rural nurses and clinic staff generally has been somewhat unwarranted. What is clear is the confusion from April to July about the support that the rural health sector would be able to provide.

The rural nurses interviewed as part of this research stated that they had received no training on how to deal with Covid-19 cases. They claimed that the health department had said that training would be provided, but it had never happened, presumably because the provincial department was thrown into crisis with the shock of the pandemic. The nurses said that they were referring patients to urban or larger rural hospitals because they did not feel trained to deal with them. It was also reported that the national Department of Health had assured regional structures that specially trained Covid-19 nurses would be deployed to the rural Eastern Cape to assist with the management of the pandemic. This measure was not well communicated;

some areas allegedly interpreted this as a statement that the existing nursing staff would lose their jobs and be replaced because they had not been trained to deal with Covid-19. Perhaps in response to these feared job losses, stories began to circulate that the trained nurses who had been promised were actually carriers of the virus; rural people were warned not to interact with them to avoid infection.

Meanwhile, a lack of medicines at rural clinics added to the perception that these institutions were ineffective at this time of need. Many respondents told us that they did not even attempt to go to the clinic, fearing that it would be a dangerous site of infection, and doubting that clinics could even be of much help. Our fieldwork revealed there was little resistance to embracing Western bio-medical treatments in the rural areas—interviewees were keen to access medication and support from the clinics. However, they found that nurses and clinics were not able to properly respond to their needs. When they did make contact, most said that they were simply referred to the city hospitals—which were generally closed.

Fear and mental health in the Eastern Cape health sector

In September 2020, Lokuthula Maphalala, a doctor at Dora Nginza Provincial Hospital in Port Elizabeth, reflected that Covid-19 was not merely a crisis of physical infrastructure, public health management and bio-medicine in the province. It was also a fundamental crisis of mental readiness and fear. She was herself not initially on the front-line, but that soon changed when her office was converted into a PPE changing room. Along with senior nurses, Dr Maphalala was tasked with repurposing wards and offices to deal with the pandemic. She explained that at the height of the pandemic they were receiving about 25 new patients a day who were in a chronic condition. Some were even already dead as their families had waited too long to bring them in. Dr Maphalala remembers that when the Covid pandemic broke out in the province, the planning process was initially chaotic. She said that they almost instantly realised that the existing emergency plan was impractical: "it was time to go back to the drawing board". This led to endless meetings and negotiations, which meant that: "it took a while before people realised that Covid-19 was here and that they had to work together."[40] One central problem was that workers, porters, doctors, and nurses seemed unable to admit that they were terrified of the Covid threat to their lives. As a result, they focused on all sort of other issues, such as broken windows and lack of equipment, to delay action and divert attention away from the main issue: fear. Maphalala believes that many of her colleagues struggled to vocalise their valid fear and anxieties: "What people needed to say was 'I am scared and I don't want to see patients'. Not being able to say those words meant that their fears and anxieties manifested as resistance to treating patients at the facility".[41]

In May 2020, Professor Zukiswa Zingela, at the Mthatha Hospital Sisonke programme in the former Transkei, led a multidisciplinary team in researching the psychosocial aspects of the pandemic. The Sisonke programme's main aim was to lend clinical and social support services to healthcare workers during this time of crisis. Accordingly, the programme focused on the fears and anxieties of health workers and allowed them to process their stress in a healthy way. Professor Zingela explained her motivation in taking this step:

> My biggest fear was that our healthcare system was not ready to address this issue. When South Africa started to brace itself for the Covid-19 storm all kinds of resources were mobilised to capacitate the healthcare system, but the one thing that was left unattended was psychosocial support for healthcare workers during this time.[42]

In the latter half of 2020, the programme grew in the province, reaching health care workers, hospitals and clinics in many parts of the rural Eastern Cape. The initiative also received some support from the provincial Department of Education. One example of the programme's work was recorded in the Engcobo area, when the organization was called in to counsel staff and community members after a health worker had stabbed a patient. The formation of this service was a direct response to the very low levels of trust that existed between health workers and communities during thw initial phases of the pandemic, and the high levels of hospital and clinic closures due to stress and fear. Professor Zingela said that it was now time: "to make mental health everybody's business, and it is as urgent for us to support our healthcare workers as it is for us to provide support to our patients".[43]

With time, Dr Maphalala also came to recognize that providing effective care was a matter of mutual respect, understanding and working together. She explained:

> It is not just about the doctors, it's everyone in the system: the cleaners, the kitchen staff, the porters, the security guards. Everyone is doing their bit and that has made all the difference.[44]

Minister Mkize and his bio-medical experts' negative and overly technical view of the province's state of readiness in April, and his public scolding of Eastern Cape Health officials, proved counterproductive in at least one respect. It instilled terror in the minds of provincial healthcare workers, who firmly believed that, due to the Eastern Cape's weak health service, they were sure to be infected and die. Many simply ran for the hills, especially those with comorbidities. Others fought with their peers and colleagues at work or found grievances that would keep them away from work and out of the firing line. There were walk-outs, strikes and absenteeism across the system. It took a long time and the rapid reduction of cases to begin to restore trust and rebuild cooperation. As infections decreased in August 2020, health workers developed better recognition of their stress and the limits of their response; they have now started to develop a more collaborative approach to managing the pandemic.

The state of Transkei hospitals: Nessy Knight and Mthatha General

Minister Mkhize openly acknowledged the deep crisis in the Eastern Cape health system on his arrival in the province in April 2020. However, he spoke in limited terms about the crisis when he stressed staff shortages at key hospitals and testing and counting inconsistencies. In June and July 2020, as the Covid crisis worsened in the province, the TAC and the Igazi Foundation wrote letters to the Department. They demanded an immediate response from the government to the untenable situation in the provincial healthcare sector. This resulted in Mkhize's second visit and his appointment of a new crisis team—lead by ministerial advisor Dr Sibongile Zungu—to assist the provincial Department and produce an assessment for Premier Oscar Mabuyane. In early July, the Premier then responded with a further set of measures and restrictions, including the declaration that all dead bodies needed to be tested for Covid and buried within three days. The Premier also promised to take steps "to address service delivery, administrative, infrastructure facility and clinical problem in some hospitals and in the provincial Department of Health in order to improve the health intervention of our response to COVID 19".[45] The striking feature of these regulations, as we pointed out in the previous chapter, was that they aggravated and compounded rural fear and panic, especially around funerals and death rituals. The attitude of the Minister and his team when managing public health was very similar. They offered top-down instructions without displaying any empathy or appreciation of the conditions in rural communities.

In August 2020, at the end of the first Covid wave, the Deputy Public Prosecutor Kholeka Gcaleka visited the region to review the reportedly dire state of rural hospitals and the failing health infrastructure, especially in the former Transkei. *Spotlight*, a public interest health sector publication, followed the senior official's visit to two hospitals in the former Transkei: Nessy Knight Hospital in Qumbu, and the Mthatha General hospital, which closed several times during June and July 2020 at the height of the first wave of the pandemic.[46] The *Spotlight* reporter wrote:

> At the Nessie Knight Hospital in Qumbu in the OR Tambo District, visibly sick patients queue for hours to consult doctors and nurses. The hospital buildings appear dilapidated, with exposed electricity cables hanging from walls and paint peeling off in places. In some wards there are broken windows and obviously damaged plumbing. Hygiene at the 80-bed district hospital has also been compromised after the laundry machine broke down recently. We understand that the hospital now has a van to ferry the laundry to other nearby hospitals to be washed.

A 2014 report on Nessie Knight Hospital had previously suggested that wide-ranging problems must be addressed as a matter of priority: poor ventilation in the ward, the disrepair of the buildings, and the nurses' accommodation in caravans. The only issues that had been addressed by August 2020 was an improvement in the accommodation situation for nurses. Nessie Knight was still flagged as a poorly performing hospital, and had received scores of less than 40% for cleanliness, patient safety and waiting times in 2016. The Deputy Public Prosecutor described the conditions at the hospital as "depressing".

At Mthatha General, Gcaleka found that the hospital had been operating without a CEO or a head of clinical services for more than a year. The *Spotlight* reporter saw patients waiting long hours in the hospital corridors due to limited space, and also noted the run-down, poorly maintained infrastructure. Social distancing was also not being properly observed. There was a desperate lack of PPE for staff working in high-risk areas, and a lack of communication from management regarding safety and well-being, which placed a heavy burden on staff.[47] The patients interviewed were indignant. Viwe Mawonga, who came to collect papers for her new-born child said: "I arrived here in the morning, but no one seems willing to assist me and it is cold out here waiting with my baby. I only want a discharge letter and proof of birth". We heard many similar stories of patients who came to collect the paperwork for death certificates, which were needed to claim funeral and life-insurance policies.

Thokozile Mhlongo, the Coordinator for the Eastern Cape Health Crisis Action Committee, raised questions about the controversial, short-run Scooter ambulances being fast-tracked in the province, when the conventional ambulance system in rural areas was virtually non-existent. In general, he noted:

> We continue to receive alarming reports from both healthcare users and the healthcare workers about the dire state of public health facilities in the province. We hold the department of health accountable because people are suffering and their dignity is being trampled on every day in public health facilities.[48]

In July 2020, Premier Oscar Mabuyane acknowledged the appalling state of affairs in terms of public health in the region, especially in the rural areas:

> For too long the rural masses of our people in particular have been receiving healthcare facilities that were not conducive for the provision of quality healthcare. Even worse, our healthcare workers had to ensure working in shabby healthcare facilities. I have seen some of these facilities with my own eyes. It still boggles the mind how they

maintained their status as healthcare facilities with their horrible state of infrastructure decay.

Premier Mabuyane said that he wanted to ensure that, after the Covid pandemic, healthcare facilities delivered a decent service and inspired hope for the people. The National Education and Allied Workers Union officials seemed sceptical. They had heard all these promises before from previous Premiers of the province, and felt that no improvement had been forthcoming. The Union also stated that corruption was rife in the department, and had been for a long time. They stated categorically that the government and the Department of Health was killing its members, and did not seem to care that so many of its health workers had died due to the poor working conditions.[49] The TAC, on the other hand, called for mobile units that could be flexibly deployed to crisis point to help relieve the pressure on the system.

Hope and improvisation at Zithulele

It is not surprising that many health workers were terrified of the frontline, given this context of great fear and vulnerability, caused by appalling urban and rural health infrastructure and the absence of protective equipment in the province, as well as the chaotic state of the provincial department. It is understandable that many developed strategies of avoidance, using whatever means they could to prevent being highly exposed to a deadly virus in an unprotected situation. The unions also had every right to support vulnerable workers. There were also protests in July that the provincial Department was using Community Health Workers (CHWs) to plug the gaps in the system, but was underpaying them and offering very limited protection from the virus. As the CHWs were in casual employment, they did not have the protection of unions and were open to abuse by a Department that was leaning heavily on these casual workers in a time of crisis.[50]

However, in the midst of rural hospital walk-outs, clinic closures and failures around the provision of ambulance services in the province, there is also no doubt that Eastern Cape health workers displayed enormous bravery and ingenuity as they tried to manage under impossible conditions. One of the most striking stories of improvisation comes from the Zithulele Hospital, a 146-bed facility in Mqanduli in the rural part of the OR Tambo district. The hospital serves around 130,000 people; like most rural hospitals in the Transkei it had to steer its own way through the Covid crisis, using whatever resources were at hand. Dr Hans Hendricks, a local family physician, and Dr Ben Gaunt, the clinical manager, recognised the limits of the facility as they began to estimate receiving a hundred new patients a day as the pandemic worsened. While their numbers thankfully never reached these levels, they had already thought through this challenge by June and were making vital changes in the hospital to get ready for this eventuality. Unlike some other rural hospitals, Zithulele luckily still had access to both water and an electricity supply in the middle months of 2020.[51]

One of the first clinical decisions made at Zithulele was to empty out the TB ward, where the number of cases had been declining, and put the remaining patients on a home-care regime. This opened up the ward for Covid patients. The second set of decisions concerned rationalising the use of limited protective equipment by classifying high and low priority areas and needs in the hospital, rather than adopting a one size fits all approach. According to Dr Gaunt, it made a difference. The hospital also made direct contact with Eskom to identify the grid on which it operated, and received assurance that they would not experience power cuts. Once all these measures had been implemented, they turned their attention to the problem of ventilation equipment. They decided to redirect, repurpose and DIY upgrade existing CPAP ventilations units from the paediatric ward to service Covid-19 patients. Dr Hendricks explained:

> Continuous Positive Airway Pressure (CPAP) [used for high-flow nasal oxygen] has been used for a very long time in paediatric wards for children with infant distress syndrome. Government has rolled out special machines for use in neonates across the country. With high flow machines initially delayed due to procurement issues, we had to see what equipment we had at the hospital and work with it to save patients.[52]

> This CPAP is a bedside device that is used to gently keep air blowing into the upper airways of the child. The doctors at Zithulele used the basis system to create their own version of the CPAP by making a

mask from a bag value mask and adding tubing connected to wall oxygen, as well as a reservoir from a non-rebreather mask and an underwater intercostal drain set. It appears that the water process helped to create pressure which forced the oxygen into the lungs through the old system, which was large passive, and thus took on the character of a mechanical ventilator.

We used the piping from the oxygen mask, an intercostal drain bottle and an anesthetic mask to mask to build the "bush CPAP" device, including duct tape and a cable-tie. The device works in the same way for kinds and adults, fitting over the mouth and nose with a seal, providing a mix of air and oxygen at a slight pressure. We made them (CPAPs) as we went along, and the device could be cleaned or sterilized and then re-used. We made about 10 of the devices.[53]

The hospital saved lives with the improvised ventilators, which most of their serious Covid patients spent several days and even weeks on. Many survived to tell the tale. The work and achievements of the doctors and staff at Zithulele now features in a special article in *African Journal of Emergency Medicine*.

Interestingly, Drs Hendricks and Gaunt confirmed that the biggest overall challenge of the Covid crisis in the rural Eastern Cape was the climate of fear that gripped the hospital and surrounding communities. Dr Hendricks said:

The biggest issue was the staff's mental health. Covid was not so bad. Some staff members were very scared. Others didn't pitch for work, and that increased the workload for those that were there. We must add that the team at the hospital is [now] very solid, although some issues at the beginning of the pandemic caused friction. As we went over the hurdle of fear, we realized that we can actually do this. It was not as bad as we thought.[54]

Dr Gaunt agreed:

Fear is actually a huge challenge. We have staff with comorbidities, so they were worried about their personal safety and that of their colleagues. The other fear was getting the virus at the hospital and taking it back into the communities and families. As this virus was new, people had little or no understanding of it. We all had to learn as we went along. I think the worst is now over.[55]

Traditional healers bridge the gap

As the state bio-medical system was unable to respond effectively to the threat of Covid-19, many households turned to traditional remedies and strategies to protect themselves against infection. In interviews conducted with traditional healers in the former Transkei, we heard that regional associations of healers had met to discuss the threat that Covid-19 posed, and had decided on some local medicines and remedies to recommend to those with symptoms. The traditional healers wished that the government had involved them in discussions about Covid-19, so that they could respond with the support of the state. One OR Tambo traditional healer stated: "if the government can allow traditional healers to operate legally and assist health official it would be better." She noted that: "it is not only Western ways that can assist during this time", saying "*kudala kwabakho izinto ezinje and okhokho bethu bazilwa izinto ezinje kungakabikho ezinto zakwa health*" (these illnesses have always been there and we can help officials). She also argued that, as healers, they could assist in making sure rituals were safe and that people were buried well, so that they "can meet with their ancestors". She said: "*sisono nje uba nina zifundiswa anizihoyi ezizinto kude kube ngumzuzu wokugqibela*" (it is a shame that educated people are not taking these things [*amasiko*, the rituals] seriously until the last minute).[56]

Other healers said that they had been called when families feared that a person had not died of natural causes and suspected evil spirits. Under these conditions they would apply *muti* (medicine) to the body to ward off evil spirits. However, the healers said that their service had no longer been required once coffins were shut by the funeral parlours and families could no longer see the body of the deceased. There was great anxiety about the state's attempts to prevent people from touching or viewing the bodies of their deceased kin, with several community members saying they would not allow the state to undermine family and cultural traditions. In one interview, this sense of defiance was expressed as follows:

> I then asked one of the family members: "*kutheni nibona umzimba nangona kungavumelekanga ukwenza lonto?*" (why did you open the casket and view when government has placed strict restrictions on such ritu-

als?). He had this to say first, "*akulawuli mapolisa apha*" (police have no jurisdictions nor authority over this family); second, "*abanye abantu bangcwabe imizimba engeyiyo eyabo ngenxa yalemithetho karhulumente*" (some families buried wrong unidentified bodies due to lockdown regulations and we could not stand that); and third, "*besifuna ukumbona okokugqibela sivalelise*" (we wanted to see her one more time and find closure before the ceremonial send-off).[57]

The traditional healers felt marginalised by the government's decision to stop customary ceremonies, which they were centrally involved in. Their main complaint was the shutting down of initiation schools and lodges (*amabhoma*) because "during this time, as a Sangoma, we would be actively involved in the initiation of young boys". They felt that "this is not possible now because many ceremonies are banned and the business of the traditional healer as custodian of cultural practises is affected." Another healer said: "I couldn't even call *intlombe* (the graduation ceremony when one becomes a traditional healer) but the person who initiated me was here, and we slaughtered a chicken. Other things will follow when the country goes back to normal."[58]

However, while the involvement of traditional healers in rituals was curtailed by the regulations, many healers stated that people were consulting them with increasing frequency because they were unwell or afraid of the virus. One healer stated:

> People come in huge numbers more than before the outbreak of Covid-19, people come from quarantine straight to *esigodlweni* because *akukho zinto bazinikwayo ezinyanga esisifo ngaphandle nje kwezinto ezimnandi* (people are not given any medication that treats or cures). This means more work and more responsibility for me. *Ndinamathwasa am kodwa ayindihluphi lonto ngoba ndabizwa ndisetyenziswa ngabantu abadala mna namathwasa am* (I have my initiates anyway and this is not a problem for me because I am called and used by the elders with my initiates). In government departments, people work eight hours, we work 15 hours a day to help people with less price in certain cases because we are afraid to chase people away unattended to in case something happened to him, and we could not assist him because of money. We assist people even if they don't have money to pay, *abanayo inkomo yegqirha* in case he dies *esigodlweni* and bring us bad luck.[59]

The healer went on to say that people came to them after leaving quarantine, as health officials had failed to provide these patients with any care.

Healers also stated that they had achieved some success in alleviating the symptoms associated with Covid-19, such as tight chests and flu symptoms. One healer said that *umhlonyane* (Artemisia Afar) and Gumtree leaves were the most common herbs now used by traditional healers. Another noted: "Even though they do not want to be identified, people who lost hope while in hospital continue to try our medicine and do recover." One traditional healer claimed to have "healed people with Covid", using *umhlonyane*. He lamented the fact that, despite his successes, the government refused to work with him. Another praised the effectiveness of *umhlonyane* saying: "*Ndicebisa abantu xa bothe iheater babeke imbiza enomhlonyane ne gumtree, ziyibetha ziyivuthulule lento*" (I advise people to place a pot with water and *umhlonyane* on the heater, while warming themselves).[60]

Another said:

Urhulumente akawahoyanga amagqirha nje tu, akawaxabisanga amagqirha at all (the government does not care about traditional practice and healers). If *amagqirha angake anikezwe chance yokuba ayosebenza esibhedlele aphathe impepho namakhandlela awo angayi identifaya cause yalento nezinye izinto ezinxulumene nale* (if traditional healers can be given a chance, they could identify the cause of this Covid-19 virus. As a traditional healer she had lost no infected patients but had cured them, whereas the Department of Health is up and down with much failure).

She added: "They not winning".[61]

One cleric from Lusikisiki explained why rural communities and families were making extensive use of local medical remedies and traditional healers:

The response of the local people from the beginning of this outbreak was negative because the government enforced regulations *without explaining the cause*. In fact, the government did not provide enough awareness on the virus, but just forced people to comply with the regulations. … the reason why they fear Corona and why the clinics are closed is the fact that no one is sure how it spreads and how it can be avoided without disturbing the lives of the people. There is just fear and misunderstanding all around. When this happens people still have their own traditional cultural beliefs and use traditional healers.[62]

Once the rural clinics started to close, rural communities asked the traditional leaders what they should do to protect themselves against the mysterious and deadly virus. In April, many communities seemed to believe that the virus was only in the cities and came from Chinese people and whites. There was even a belief that blacks would not be infected. There were Chinese traders in the rural towns in the Transkei, so people avoided them for good measure. After Easter 2020, when migrants came home from the cities, the idea that only whites and Asians could contract the virus faded. People started to fear outsiders from the urban areas, including members of their own families. The older folks in the village suggested that home-comings should be monitored with caution, although there was no loss of enthusiasm for family members attending funerals. The fear of funerals came much later in the year, as we will see in chapter six. In a climate of uncertainly and spiritual insecurity, people turned to traditional leaders for advice. They were told to use tried and tested family remedies and to consult traditional healers. One respondent from Goso Village in Encgobo said:

> The traditional leaders advise people to use the natural herbs like "*Umhlonyane*" and "gumtree" leaves, which if steamed can heal cold and flu… People saw Mr Z. Vavi who recovery from Covid-19. He advises people to also use "*umhlonyane*" for healing. It grows near the river and can be dug out with ease. People grew up using it in old days. There people are now trying by all means to get and use natural herbs. Traditional leaders are trying to communicate about the Covid-19, but so far families are doing it on their own with herbs like *umhlonyane* and gumtree leaves. This is also because the clinics are closed.[63]

One of the traditional healers we interviewed confirmed this trend and also highlighted some of the techniques he used:

> As clinics close in most of the Transkei, rural people were encouraged by chiefs and healers on the use of indigenous plants. They already know and have been using for fever and flu related symptoms. I am a healer, and I am treating 6 Covid patients right now. I find that the secret to success is in the mixing of the herbs and the specific timing

of giving the concoctions to the patient, so that medicinal elements can be drawn from the plant. The most relevant organic plants for this mixture can also be revealed to me in dreams, especially when patients are having problems. I learnt that the herb *umhlonyane* is best boiled or burned for Covid to draw its scent. Making it into a juice for treatment of covid related symptoms is best. The same with gum-tree leaves. I am finding that my treatments are now curing Covid-19, and many people are now coming to me for help.[64]

Abandoned communities

The state's immediate response following the declaration of the Covid-19 lockdown in the rural Eastern Cape was to crack down on customary ceremonies and practices. As well as calling on rural communities to comply with government regulations, police swept through these areas to stop customary practices which had been categorised as unlawful. This campaign riled the rural poor, who felt they had hardly been made aware of the regulations before the police were destroying their possessions and undermining their customary rights. The repressive police campaign, supported by traditional leaders, left a bitter taste in the mouths of many rural residents. They felt that the police were overzealous and that the rules had not been properly communicated. Meanwhile, the entire Eastern Cape government was thrown into disarray as it failed to keep its hospitals and public buildings clean and provide its workers with PPE. The public sector unions went on strike as a result.

The furore started at Zwide clinic in Port Elizabeth, which had been serving 500 people each day. The absence of deep cleaning and PPE led to infections among the nursing staff, who then walked out with the support of their union. They refused to return to work until standard operating procedures were implemented and the facility was properly cleaned. This episode set the stage for multi-institutional shutdowns across the province; dozens of government service providers from Home Affairs offices, to hospitals and police stations closed. Once shuttered, it could take anything from a few days to a month for the facilities to re-open. Meanwhile, the services were suspended as frontline workers languished at home. The scale of institutional shutdown was great. Almost every government department providing face-to-face services suffered closures at one point, from the post offices to the most remote rural clinics. Rural communities who were already living in fear—of the unknown; of infection; of the police; of returning migrants; and of crowds at funerals—were offered no reassuring presence by the state. Indeed, the state and some senior traditional leaders were conspicuous by their absence.

This chapter has focused on the conditions at rural hospitals and clinics. It detailed how nurses were especially nervous of infection and reluctant to put their lives on the line, having received little or no training or Covid-19-related instruction. The rural hospitals and clinics were also late in receiving PPE and were increasingly under pressure as infections spiked in rural areas from June. There were a number of doctor and nurse walk-outs in small rural hospitals, as well as dozens of rural clinics that closed their doors due to lack of equipment and instruction. The promised arrival of Covid-19 trained nurses, Cuban doctors and South African Defence Force personnel to alleviate the situation never materialised. In this environment of generalised fear and confusion, we found that rural communities and households were left to improvise and fall back on indigenous knowledge systems to assist their physical and psychological resistance to the pandemic. Our fieldwork research found that large numbers of rural households were making regular use of medicinal plants, including gum leaves and *umhlonyane*, and were buying locally produced Covid-19 concoctions brewed by local healers. At the same time, traditional healers, who had been marginalised by the ban on customary practices, complained bitterly that the government had failed to include them in their plans to manage the pandemic in rural areas. In general, the situation pointed to a lack of coordination and integration between formal and informal healthcare systems, and among the different governance structures in the rural areas.

4

DIVIDED HOMESTEADS

Introduction

On 19 March 2020, the Indian Railways announced that they would suspend all passenger trains across the country due to the rising Covid crisis. The Indian government declared a national lockdown to control the spread of the pandemic. The announcement created panic in a country where, especially in urban areas, a significant portion of the workforce are bona fide migrants. Perhaps as much as a third of Indians make their livings by circulating between small rural farms and the cities. Migrants dominate in the informal sector, which employs over 90% of the Indian workforce. Many in this sector vacillate between low paid work in the cities, often under inhuman conditions, and some form of subsistence farming on the land. In the migrant livelihood strategies, the "source village" serves as an anchor for coping, as the land supports many in the migrant family. There are regional variations in the patterns of movement, work cycles and relative importance of "source" and "destination" sites, but most migrants still depend on opportunities at both ends of the urban-rural spectrum. They construct trans-local livelihoods by moving seasonally between town and countryside. The implementation of lockdown in India and the closure of passenger rail, the preferred transport system, created panic in the migrant community. Their first instinct,

115

when the streets emptied and the informal economy ground to a halt, was to return to the rural areas, as they would not be able to survive in the cities without income. This produced mass reverse migration in India with profound implications for the rural areas, which received hundreds of thousands of returning migrants from the cities who had lost their income.

In May 2020, following graphic images and stories in the media of Indian migrants making their way home on foot, Ajay Dandekar and Rahul Ghai wrote in the *Economic and Political Weekly*:

> In the last few weeks, we have all been witness to harrowing, nerve wrenching and bone chilling images of the exodus of marginal and "invisible" [migrants] drivers of the informal economy of urban India. Indian highways emptied of most vehicles were lined with bedraggled poor pedestrians, many carrying all their worldly belongings in bundles on the top of their heads walking to their home villages, hundred or thousands of miles away across states. Add to that equally desperate attempts by small distance migrants to somehow reach their (home) destinations from medium sized towns and cities and we have a scenario of crowded back villages that constitute the famished and dried up "source". Even as this is written, there are field reports emerging about the scarcity of food and water compounding the dried source. The crop harvest.... will provide some relief in the short run, but the sources regions cannot be relied on to take the additional load of the returning sons and daughters of the region.[1]

Ajay Dandekar and Rahul Ghai called for a charter of rights to protect migrants. The Indian government responded by setting measures and protections to support migrants, and eventually supported over 600,000 migrants to return home. Similar processes occurred in other parts of the world, especially in relation to transnational migrants. In South Africa, provisions were made for Zimbabwean migrants to return home in large numbers at the end of March 2020, but there was less discussion about the management of the internal migration dynamic within the country.[2]

In the South African informal settlements and townships, the human economy of migrant labour differed from the situation in India because urban and rural livelihoods were less intertwined after apartheid. This was partly because the post-apartheid welfare social system provided a source of cash income to rural households that was not dependent on their connections with kin in the cities. By 2010, almost 70% of all rural households in South Africa received some sort of grant, such as pension, disability, or child support. While this could not cover the full cost of social reproduction in these areas, it did make families much less dependent on migrant remittances. There were also more opportunities for urban stabilisation, if households could get access to subsidised state low-cost housing. However, urban migrants faced very limited opportunities for informal earning in towns and cities because of the stagnation of the industrial economy after apartheid. The formal, large-scale retail and supermarket sector entered the townships and rural areas with malls and cheap products that soaked up wages and social grants. This meant that the informal sector struggled to grow, while existing black small business created under apartheid in ethnic enclaves crumbled.[3] In South Africa, the urban and the rural were thus less closely interlocked at the level of everyday livelihood-making. However, they were closely intertwined in other ways: the welfare grants supported the children of many migrants, and the homestead where ancestors resided remained both an anchor for family identities and an escape from the precarity and violence of everyday urban life. Family pride and identity also remained tied to rural homesteads. After apartheid, these were often reconstructed as modern suburban homes rather than old-fashioned farmsteads, as increasing numbers of household members migrated to the cities in search of work. In this context, the old colonial and apartheid patterns of returning home to plough over Christmas, or reaping the harvest at Easter, were much less pronounced, even though agrarianism has remained a valued element in the construction of rural family identities.[4]

When the Coronavirus broke out in South Africa in March 2020, and it was becoming clear that the country would be entering a lockdown, the South African government created a small window of opportunity for migrants to travel home. The measures seemed to be created mainly with international travellers and migrants in mind. However, in the informal settlements of Cape Town, many recalled this period of animated debate, especially amongst the families with connections to homes in the Eastern Cape. Sanele, from Imizamo Yethu township in Hout Bay, Cape Town, recalled:

People were talking about going home, and their first feeling was to think that if there was to be a catastrophe, they would want to be at home with their families. If you are going to die in our culture, it is better to die at home. But they also worried about losing their place in the township.... Once you give up your shack or room here, it is not easy to get it back. Township landlords tend to be ruthless. They rent to the highest bidder these days and poor migrants can lose out to foreigners with money. When people lost their jobs, they were out and could not survive, so they had to move somewhere, like moving to a sister or uncle elsewhere in the city or going home. These were the things people were weighing up at that time.

Sanele went on to state that many people in his migrant neighbourhood with close connections to the Transkei went home—between 10 to 20% of those living in the yards and the shacks. The rest stayed behind hoping that they could still get work or hold onto their jobs, while others moved to other townships in the city. Around Easter time 2020, when the fear of the Coronavirus had taken hold, the Premier of the Eastern Cape complained that too many people from the Western Cape were flooding back into the Eastern Cape. He said that they threatened to bring the urban virus into peaceful and healthy communities in the rural Eastern Cape. He suggested that the Western Cape government of the Democratic Alliance, the official opposition to the ruling African National Congress, was deliberately not controlling outmigration to shift the burden of the pandemic to the Eastern Cape, where the government had taken decisive action to minimise the risk in rural areas by shutting down funerals and customary practices.

In September 2021, Dorrit Posel and Daniela Casale from Wits University published the results of a migration and living arrangements study, based on over 7,000 telephonic interviews between March and May 2020. Their data suggests that one in six adults in South Africa—between five and six million people—changed homes during this period, either between urban and rural areas or within urban areas. Of those who moved household, 82% made one move, while 18% moved more than once. The authors also suggest that at the time of Covid about 20% of all households in South Africa were migrant households or stretched households, where at least one member was absent for at least four to five nights a week. But there is also a difference between active economic circular migration in South Africa and "double-rootedness". Under double-rootedness, members of rural households have effectively left for the cities to work, but are not seen as absentees because they remain connected to their rural homes, which they aim to rebuild and hope to return to. In other words, many more of those living in the cities retained the option of rural return, or "reverse migration" in South Africa, than the 20% of so-called "migrant or stretched households". Posel and Casale also argue that, while around a third of those in stretched households were in poverty before 2020, their data suggests this number increased to almost half after March 2020. This suggests that South Africa also experienced a wave of reverse migration during the first Covid wave, which placed pressure on rural households. The aim of this chapter is to explore the growing tensions, fear and struggles behind the garden gate in rural homesteads during the first lockdown period from April to July 2020.[5]

Home-coming and the Easter harvest

When this research began in April and May 2020, households were harvesting their annual garden crops across the Transkei. Families who had planted maize in the latter part of 2019 were bringing in their crop from homestead gardens and fields. There was some excitement across the region because the yields looked encouraging. In the rural Transkei, the harvest has historically been an extended social event, starting around April with the harvesting of green maize from gardens, and running through until the end of July. Unripened green maize is used to feed animals and even families if there is hunger, before the harvest officially starts. In every location where this study was conducted, the researchers noticed piles of mealies which had been gathered standing outside homesteads.[6] In the past, homesteads would make use of fields and gardens, but since the 1950s homestead production was largely confined to small homestead gardens, especially since the male labour that would do the ploughing was now away working on the mines. Homestead gardening could nevertheless be extremely productive, especially if the soils were rich and families intercropped maize, pumpkins, potatoes and other vegetables. Intermittent drought and migrancy always negatively impacted the capacity of families to produce crops on the land, and most surveys showed that with further youth outmigration since the end of apartheid, only around one in three rural households were actively using their garden. However, when the rains were good, as was the case in 2019, more families found the wherewithal to plant, as is evidenced by the harvest of April 2020.

On this issue, agrarian specialist Paul Hebinck states that social scientists tend to see social change in the Eastern Cape countryside in linear terms, such as a singular shift from farming to non-farming; from agriculture to wage labour; from wages to welfare dependence; or even from adherence to traditional culture to modernity.[7] He challenges this view by suggesting that homes and households are always in a cycle of activation and de-activation. This causes changes, not only during the course of the year, but over the longer term as their membership and livelihood strategies shift. The household life-cycle has an impact on these changes and the needs of rural families change.[8] But Hebinck also suggests that, in terms of local cultural orientation, it is not possible or desirable to shut a rural homestead down completely because that would cut the family off from its spiritual connections to the ancestors—so homesteads are always being reactivated, re-agrarianised or resuscitated.[9] The assertion here is also that Xhosa culture cannot easily exist outside the rural, agrarian imagination, however urbanised it might become.[10] In exploring the impacts of the spread of the Coronavirus in the former Transkei between April and August 2020, the above insights are important general context for an assessment of household- and community-level responses.

Figure 4 highlights the current focus of investment in the rural areas. In this image, we see how a small rectangular rural house (on the right) has been upgraded and modernised into a suburban-style home with a gabled entrance. In all these sites it is important to note here that the traditional round houses, which used to have thatched rooves in the past, and other outbuildings, including storage facilities and cattle byres are seldom removed. This is because, despite the current focus on the modernisation of the family house, families require these facilities for family rituals, animal sacrifice and agrarian pursuits, like storing maize. The status of families in the rural landscape today depends a great deal on the size, look and suburban feel of the family house, which has become a symbolic representation of the family's ability to improve its standing in the new democracy. In the cities, migrants and newly urbanised families often have access to little more than tin shacks, or a backyard room, so the integrity of the family home in the rural areas is often a priority and a matter of joint family concern. For poorer household with limited means, even just having a pile of bricks in the rural yard can show the intent to "improve", urbanise and display a more consumerist orientation, even if the family has not yet managed to lay the foundations of an improved home. These neighbourhood developments attract attention when friends and family return home for the cities for funerals and other rituals, or at Christmas and Easter time. Thabo from the Idutywa area remarked that:

> This house renovation thing is completely out of hand in the rural areas now, everyone is looking around to see what others are doing. They are comparing what others are doing to what they have. It is undermining the old sense of community when people had round houses that were all the same. In those days they would see how many cattle a family had or judge them by the size of the maize yield. Things are different today, it is all about the size and shape of the house, and how modern it looks and how many pillars are around the front door.[11]

Thabo explained that many people cluster their homes in the main family site rather than seek their own separate plots with gardens. New families often do this because they are looking for work in the cities and do not have enough people at home to maintain a new homestead. Others explained that this tendency was a product of a dramatic drop in marriage rates, which meant that adult family members were still effectively part of their parental homestead. The clustering of dwellings in a single site was also beneficial because it meant that there would always be someone at home to tend to the homestead and plant the garden while others were away. The idea of a homestead being active and committed to community, Thabo said, was often expressed through involvement in traditional activities such as farming the land and raising livestock or chickens. These activities keep the "garden gate open" and signal a commitment to participating in the community.

Although small-scale farming in the region has diminished over the years, and rural areas have been gripped by new forms of consumerism and identity, in 2020 a sizeable minority of households still accessed food from their gardens and fields. The coincidence of the spread of Covid-19 and the time of harvesting was thus significant. The outbreak happened as locally produced food was made available to support households and shared among neighbours and kin. For example, a community member in Lusikisiki stated, "during the harvest time, we got assistance from our neighbours, and we help each other out as community members. In return, we will give out food that we harvested to others to use at home". One of the chiefs explained: "People in the rural area, are people who are helping each other. When one does not have salt, he goes and asks for it next door, but now because of this pandemic people are no longer allowed to go next door."[12] He said that the fear of Coronavirus would affect the rural communal spirit of sharing, based on the African philosophy of *ubuntu*. Others said that the idea of community was over-emphasised by traditional leaders and old folks, and that those who harvested from their gardens and fields usually had to pay people to work or hire a tractor to help plough the fields and cart the produce. This was different from the old spirit of work parties and locally organised ploughing teams. Many said that special events—funerals and rituals, or home-comings at Easter and Christmas—were the catalysts for community spirit and cooperation today, rather than bringing in the maize harvest. Traditionally, surplus maize was converted into beer at harvest time, which encouraged social interaction and made harvest a good time for neighbourly and family rituals.

In contrast to the stereotype old and new, Eastern Cape scholar Zolani Ngwane has noted that the Xhosa homestead is far less cohesive than many anthropologists have assumed.[13] He argues that rural homesteads mainly unite in adversity and during certain times of the year, like Easter and Christmas, when family members are eager to return from the city. In the first half of the 20th century, when more agrarian production was undertaken on the land, these visits were often extended, especially during the summer planting season when men had to drive the oxen used for ploughing. Women could manage and maintain gardens and even guide the harvest, but they were not supposed to drive the cattle. Ngwane argues that between Easter and Christmas rural households were often socially thin and vulnerable as people struggled for survival and moved away to the cities.[14] He quotes lyrics from the famous Eastern Cape jazz band, the Blue Notes, which suggest that people do their own thing and fight with each other as they head for the cities, until they return home for Christmas. Social relations and cohesion in rural households and communities thus seem to wax and wane over the year. Nevertheless, the period between April and July is usually one of greater optimism and sociality as families reunite at Easter and start preparing for the harvest in June.

When the pandemic arrived just before Easter 2020, rural families were therefore expecting migrants to come home. They were just starting to harvest, which implied sharing food and social activity. But rural communities at this time also feared that urban migrants would bring the dreaded virus with them; many still believed that it came from China or was brought by the whites. Others said that there was no need to worry because the virus that could not be easily contracted by black people. The political discourse in April was that the rich urbanised provinces should not impose a further burden on the poor rural provinces by sending home people who were sick and dangerous. The story within individual families differed as we heard many cases where rural relatives were encouraging their urban kin to come home for Easter. In Cape Town's townships, there was a strong desire amongst migrants, as in many other parts of the world, to return home. Phila from Langa township told us that the taxis were full, and people were leaving in their droves; "not as many as in the past, but there was still a strong desire amongst people to go home for the Easter weekend". He did notice, however, that not everyone returned to the city after the weekend. "People decided to stay behind, some because they intended to go home, others stayed on because they could not get back to the city under lockdown conditions".

In the Engcobo area we heard stories of youths and women staying at home, some with children under the care of their mothers in the rural areas. It was clear from several interviews that those in the rural areas were hoping that their kin would return to the urban areas to support themselves and look for jobs. In more than one case, older women and men said that they were struggling to get by on their welfare payments and the little they could eke out of their gardens. "I am not sure how we will survive now with extra people on the same income", one woman explained. Another said: "there is no work here for the youngsters, the harvest work is done and there are no jobs in the locations, we just hope they can find piece work to help out". These responses were often accompanied by statements of relief that family members could be away from the urban frontline and would be more protected at home. Attitudes toward return migration hardened in May and June when some of the rural districts in the Eastern Cape were declared national Covid hotspots. The government blamed funerals as the main "super spreaders" in rural areas, while locals said that migrants were finding other ways to get home and bringing the disease with them. A study undertaken by Stats South Africa in June 2020 found that 15% of the random sample of people contacted indicated that they had crossed provincial borders since lockdown began in March. Of that grouping, only 25% had travelled to rural areas for funerals, which the government say are the main cause of rural transmission. The remaining 75% had travelled home for other reasons, most of which the survey was unable to determine.

In support of this ethnographic evidence, quantitative surveys from April to July suggest that spatial inequalities between urban and rural areas deepened during the first wave of Covid-19. The evidence from the NIDS-CRAM surveys shows that all communities suffered during level 5 hard lockdown in April 2020. This included middle-class suburban areas in the big cities, where significant job losses were recorded. When South Africa went down to level 4 in May, the situation improved in the suburbs, but not in the urban townships and shack areas.[15] Turok and Visagie were struck by the clearly widening gap between urban and rural areas. In the latter households are heavily dependent on social grants. Between January and June 2020, the South African government paid out R40 billion or around $3 billion in social welfare grants to rural households, who were also able to access Covid assistance at a higher rate than households in the cities.[16] Nevertheless—and partly because of reverse migration—rural households showed the highest level of food insecurity, poverty, and hunger. In the metropolitan areas, around 40% of households said that

Diagram 1: Survey of travel habits during lockdown, June–July 2020

More than a quarter (25.6%) of respondents indicated that they crossed provincial boundaries to attend funerals.

Percentage distribution of respondents who travelled across provincial boundaries during lockdown by reason for intra-provincial travel.

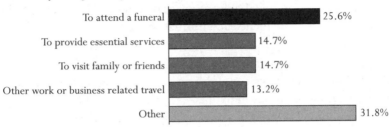

Based on data from "Social impact of COVID-19 (Wave 3): Mobility, Migration, and Education in South Africa", Department of Statistics, South Africa, 4 July 2020. Available at: http://www.statssa.gov.za/publications/Report-00-08-04/Report-00-08-04July2020.pdf

they ran out of money to buy food in April 2020, while around 55% of those in rural areas were in this position. However, this was mitigated by some crop production in rural communities. The most remarkable fact was perhaps that, between April and July 2020, one in three households rural households reported that members had gone hungry over the past seven days—almost twice as many as metropolitan urban households, where one in six had reported the same fact.[17]

Moral communities and rural realities

African scholarship makes a distinction between "wealth in things" and "wealth in people" in settings where customary power has been reconstituted during and after colonialism.[18] In pre-colonial Africa, land was abundant and human labour scarce. Scholars thus argued that controlling the "means of domination", and having power over the people, was more important than controlling land and technology, or the "means of production". A contrast can be observed between the territorial fluidity of polities in Africa, characterised by what one scholar called "snowball states",[19] and the history of Europe. In Europe, struggles over specific territories and land dominated, lead-

125

ing to a particular trajectory in the rise of nationalism. This has led to theories that African social relations are orientated towards controlling rights in people, rather than rights in things. Systems of power at the local level were connected to age, gender and status, or clan lineages or genealogies, which determined relations of dependence, social hierarchy and social obligation. Activating and honouring these relationships of dependence and mutual obligation, especially among neighbours and kin, was more important than simply holding land or changing technology. For this reason, questions have been raised about rights-based laws and public discourse which promotes self-actualising, autonomous individuals as an ideological foundation for development in Africa. The concern is particularly pertinent in rural South Africa, where the terms of the new Constitution of 1994 conflict with older regimes of generational and gender-based forms of power and dependence.[20]

In the rural Transkei, local notions such as *ubuntu*—realising one's humanity through wholesome relations of mutuality with other people—highlight people's interconnection and mutual dependence. As once community member notes, even in the time of death, "when someone dies in the community, we would just contribute whatever one has as neighbours in the society. Before Covid this was possible but since the outbreak, this has become totally impossible for me." Kathleen Rice argues that the sense of different kinds of moral obligations is expressed in the distinction people make between ideas like *amalungelo* (rights), *abantu* (people) and *irhayti* (the Xhosa word for rights derived from the English term, "rights").[21] The term *amalungelo* is derived from the verb *ukulungisa*, which mean to make things nice, correct and good in the moral sense. The term is used to highlight the moral content of personhood, especially "moral rightness" in relation to kin.[22] The critical point about the difference between *irhayti*—the individual rights reflected in the liberal discourse of the South African Constitution—and *amalungelo* is that the latter does not assume that all individuals do or should enjoy the same rights. Obligations, freedoms and rights are believed to be necessarily structured by social hierarchies of gendered and generational power.[23] The sense of community in rural areas is shaped by a matrix of expectations and aspirations related to the maintenance of a social order based on *ubuntu* and *umalungelo*. Over the past 25 years, the acquisition of political rights and the adoption of a rights-based political discourse and Constitution have challenged traditional ideas about the social order in many rural areas. This has led to the internalisation of different understandings of personhood, especially among women and youth. Young women villagers now claim that they have individual rights as citizens which cannot be brushed aside by older women and men, who appeal to past forms of gender and generational power. These women often seek to express their independence and social autonomy by providing for their families and building their careers.[24]

In this sense, the old image of the homestead as a haven of social cohesion and consensus, where everyone has a common understanding of the world, is no longer the case. In fact, the idea of what the homestead should mean in contemporary South Africa—and the roles and responsibilities of the family within it—is a matter of constant debate and contestation. Rights, duties and obligations are under review in a context of poverty, violence and inequality. Rural households should therefore not be viewed as havens from a heartless world. The extent and intensity of gender-based violence across South Africa indicates that households are not necessarily safe spaces for those who live in them. It would be wrong to think that rural households represent exceptions to this dynamic, just because they are out of sight in the former homelands. Interpersonal violence is not only an urban phenomenon in South Africa. In urban informal settlements in Cape Town, we found that young women were often the least keen to return home for visits and holidays, especially if they did not have children staying within their parental homestead in the rural areas. Many young women in service jobs in the city with secure accommodation said they were enjoying their newfound freedoms too much to return home to be bossed around by men and older women. As women got older and had families, their attitudes towards return migration changed. Even in the rural areas, young women who did not migrate to the larger cities often moved away to local small towns during the week where they worked as streets traders or sought casual employment. They would return home at the end of the week or the month to assist their parents with childcare and household chores. Women who travelled longer distances tended to see their children less frequently. The graphic below represents the contrast between the population pyramid of a rural location near in Willowvale area in the Mbashe municipality and that of Imizamo Yethu, or Mandela Park, in Hout Bay, as recorded in the 2011 national census.[25] The graphic shows that the many children stay behind in the rural homestead when their parents migrate. It also shows how female migration to the cities has increased since the end of apartheid.[26]

Diagram 2: Contrasting population pyramid of a Transkei village (*left*) in the Mbashe municipality and Cape Town shack settlement (*right*), 2011[27]

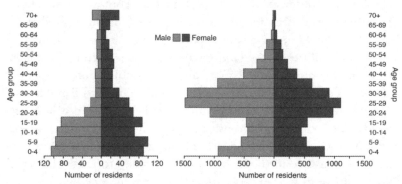

Based on data from Katherine Hall. 2017. *Children's spatial mobility and household transitions: A study of child mobility and care arrangements in the context of maternal migration.* PhD thesis, University of the Witwatersrand, Johannesburg.

By the turn of the millennium, Zolani Ngwane was right to highlight that rural households were fragmented. They are clearly sites of contested agendas and struggles over people and resources. However, this does not mean that the romantic idea of rural family coherence and healthy communities does not exist in the popular imagination, or that rural home-comings are not greeted with a sense of nostalgia. There is a yearning for a more coherent sense of community and identity, which seems to have slipped away; for a time—even if an imagined one—when there was more agreement and hope. And yet despite the decreasing optimism and rising nostalgia for the "bad old days" of homeland rule, there is still persistent hope in rural areas, waxing and waning over time. In the cycle of any year, as in the cycle of any life, there are periods in rural communities of greater sociality, sharing and community interaction, as well as periods when people feel more isolated. The concepts of *amalungelo* (mutual dependence) and *iriaythi* (individual autonomy) coexist and are expressed in different ways at different times. The period between April and the end of June (as well as the period over Christmas) is a time when Xhosa-speaking people from the Transkei region say that the "gate is open". This is a time when sharing, mutual dependence and obligation are heightened in everyday life, and people do things together, such as harvesting the crops, getting ready for the home-coming of migrants and preparing the villages for the winter male initiation rituals. In many parts of the Transkei, including large parts of Pondoland, the period of June and July is known as the initiation season, when male youths "go to the bush" to become men. Youths from villages and cities come home to the rural locations to undertake their training in preparation for manhood. As part of their transition to manhood, they are circumcised in the forests. It is a hugely important time for Xhosa-speaking communities. Boys are assembled in groups with their parents and relatives to participate in the preparations and rituals associated with male initiation, which ultimately ends with the circumcised youth returning from the bush for a massive welcoming party and ceremony back in the village.[28] Conventionally, the organisation of male initiation ceremonies coincides with harvesting and beer-brewing. It is a time of intensified social interaction, when social relations between community members thicken and local people work together in the community.

Gender and generational struggles behind the gate

The declaration of a national state of disaster from March 2020 ensured that the customary social opening of rural communities in the Transkei did not happen at Easter. The hard lockdown at the end of March saw strict measures preventing citizens from leaving their neighbourhoods, suburbs, villages and homes. The state provided a brief window for families to move to a new place for the long-term lockdown. The main aim was to allow South African citizens caught overseas to return and to permit Africans from other countries to leave. At the same time, the measure also allowed people in South Africa with two homes to decide whether they wanted to lock-down in the cities, the country-side, or their beach house. The regulations did not permit migrants to travel freely between urban and rural areas at Easter. This meant that urban residents with links to rural areas had to choose either to stay in the city or to return to their rural homes.

Given the high levels of uncertainty about the job market and employment, most migrants decided to stay in the city, despite the dangers of being locked down in overcrowded townships or informal settlements. It seems that many felt that, if they left for the safety of the countryside, they might lose access to a place in the city. Those in rental accommodation or in the backyards of township houses clearly felt that they would be replaced with other tenants. The window of opportunity came and went with only a relatively small number of migrants leaving the cities and returning home.[29] Across ten locations in eight rural municipalities,[30] there was little evidence of the home-coming anticipated over the Easter period. The situational reports from the districts showed that there was some influx into the rural areas from the cities at the end of March, when citizens were given a week to decide where they wanted to live. This late March trickle was then augmented with an additional influx over Easter as taxi drivers from Cape Town and Johannesburg made special arrangements to use roads to get people home. This was a high-risk strategy as the state was clearly willing to crack down on those breaking the law. Taxi drivers and their passengers risked receiving heavy fines and jail sentences for their efforts. Some who made the journey decided not to return after the weekend for fear of arrest. Social media videos and photographs of queues taxi ranks and convoys passing key points nevertheless revealed that taxi owners were prepared to take the risk because they needed the business.

As people arrived from the city, rural communities were accusing the government of "closing the gate" on them by shutting down funerals and customary practices. In relation to traditional ceremonies, the traditional leaders in the province took a strong stance, arguing for compliance. Rural communities were less convinced. Many felt that the state was over-reacting and undermining their cultural and family rights. They argued that small modifications of social behaviours would allow traditional gathering and customary practices to go ahead relatively safely. The one-size-fits-all approaches adopted by the state and the house of traditional leaders felt insensitive and draconian to them, and shutting everything down without even a community meeting seemed unreasonable. For these reasons, they felt justified in defying the blanket ban issued by the house of traditional leaders. In the more remote communal areas, this study's researchers found that customary practices continued openly during lockdown, as boys went to the bush as planned. The traditional surgeons and organisers of these events said that since these events had taken place in the mountains and forests, far from the settlements, it was unlikely that they would pose a threat to health. However, they were concerned about the visibility of the "home-coming" ceremonies, although they thought the restrictions would probably have been lifted by then.

When field workers started asking questions about Coronavirus in May 2020, many in the rural areas doubted that it could even kill black Africans. People were more careful about complying with regulations, such as wearing masks or physical distancing, when they felt that police might be watching or that other members of the community might report them for breaking the rules. The evidence suggests that compliance was mainly a response to fear of arrests and fines; many said that they did not follow the same rules in the villages where there was less visible law enforcement. However, the laissez-faire attitude expressed in the early days of the outbreak started to change by the end of May and into June, when certain rural districts in the Eastern Cape, such as Chris Hani and OR Tambo, were declared national Covid-19 hotspots. Families started to feel the deadly presence of the virus more directly in their neighbourhoods. What had initially been perceived as a problem for whites and Asians and subsequently a problem for the major metropolitan areas, like Cape Town and Gauteng, was now present across the Eastern Cape, where hospitals were closing and people were dying.

At this point, rural household themselves started to proactively physically distance and isolate themselves. New rumours and stories emerged about how the virus spread or could be spread in the rural setting. It was recognised that the older generation was exposed to the greatest risk, and the old started to "close the gate" in their own homesteads. They tried to impress on household members that leaving the household, or homestead precinct, was dangerous. They asked younger members not to mingle in the village, at the shops, or on the streets in towns, saying this could be deadly, especially for the old and the sickly whose welfare grants were often underpinning the economic survival of the family. The demands of the elderly were not always respected by the youth, causing tension within households. According to one community leader: "During level 5 of the national lockdown, people did not care about the outbreak, especially youth. Only elderly people were more frightened by the outbreak." As a result, "youth do not really fear Corona more than other diseases as they see it as a flu that will eventually go away".

Across all the ten communities, as the lockdown levels were lowered, concern was expressed about the youth not observing any of the rules. When alcohol went on sale again there was concern it would exacerbate youth negligence. Even though community members were unhappy about the police presence in their neighbourhoods, elderly people called for more law enforcement to check youths' reckless behaviour and enforce the regulations. Several respondents urged a return to level 5 lockdown, saying the law should be rigid. They sought more visible enforcement, including by soldiers, who were more feared than the police. They said that the only people who showed little fear of the virus a were the youth, because they believed that it only harmed older people. Even under level 5, youths were playing football with no physical distancing and without wearing masks; they would still touch each other as though nothing had changed. Police officials continually tried to change their behaviour: "*ngekungenjalongo uba bebeyoyika le corona aba bantwana*" (it wouldn't be that way if they were not afraid of this corona these children). People felt that the youth knew about the virus and its impacts, but did not care. The need to protect livelihoods and mobility in a time of crisis was given priority.

One respondent noted that "the youth who consume alcohol always say and believe that the virus only kills people who do not drink and not people who drink. *abalali ulutsha, ubusuku nemini ngo sisi, ngo bhuti ngoba bathi ayibenzinto bona ingakumbi xabesele*. (The youth does not sleep, both genders, and they believe that they will not get infected since they drink.) They do not even put on their masks." Elderly people felt that they understood and feared the Coronavirus more than the youth. A common view was that elderly people always fear death, but youth simply said "*zifa zitofile*" (no matter what you do, when death comes, it comes).

In the struggle by household heads and senior members to "close the gate", the tensions between *amalungelo* and *irhayti* were in evidence, with the youth claiming that the older generation had no place telling them what to do. They insisted that things had changed since the days of apartheid when the old women and men could just tell young people what they would do and when they would do it. They argued that they had certain freedoms, such as the freedoms of movement and association, which they were now used to and would not compromise. The rural youth argued that there now seemed to be some unholy alliance between the older generation and the state—and that both were unreasonably trying to assert control. The interviews also indicate the considerable concern of older men and women that the youth were being irresponsible and putting their lives at risk. They wanted more state and police intervention in the villages to enforce the regulations on physical distancing, and keep everyone indoors and out of the public space. As one elderly community member said:

> Deployment of police and soldiers in the community will make a difference. The lockdown regulations [should be] tightened especially in our villages. The ban of alcohol must remain because people turn not to care when they are drunk. The youth in particular does not take this virus very seriously, hence now the police must go out and monitor them and, if needs be, arrest them. The police have had to ask for assistance from the headman or councillor because of the remoteness of the area. The youth sees the police van from a distance and they start running.

The threat was believed to escalate greatly when the youth went to towns to socialise. The older generation felt that moving around in the villages was dangerous enough, without the additional risk incurred when people went to town. According to one local councillor:

> If we can go back to level 5 of lockdown and the social grants taken back to rural areas because it is easy to control few people. Mthatha

is overcrowded because people from neighbouring towns, for example, Tsolo, Mqanduli, Libode and Port St. Johns come at the times of getting social grants.

Community stakeholders have noted that when people went to town it was difficult for them to adhere to the regulations. One said: "When people are going shopping, they do not practice much social distancing outside the shops and only practice it inside because there are people watching them." It was also indicated that physical distancing was impossible on the drive into town and that people would only put on their masks when approaching areas with police. Older generation household members insisted that the youth had no right to put their lives in danger by taking such dangerous trips.

Tensions also escalated as households were locked down in a single space and members were immobile. Contestation over expected household roles and responsibilities now came to the fore.[31] The older generation appealed to the lexicon of moral femininity in this situation, expecting younger women to do the bulk of the work of caring for others and making efforts to prevent the spread of the virus. During funerals, the young women were expected to prepare the home for visitors by cleaning, cooking and serving visitors. Figures 1 and 6 show young women performing their roles during a funeral, cooking outside even in the cold; serving people in the open air; and making and serving tea for the group of people who arrive at the home of the bereaved family. Their efforts to maintain their distance, which can be observed in Figure 6, may be seen as a sign of *ukuhlonipha* (obedience). In many parts of the Transkei, women's obedience was traditionally expressed through *hlonipha* respect customs, which impressed on young women the need to behave meekly, speak softly and infrequently, carry themselves submissively and remain close to the homestead unless chaperoned. Older men and women were often proud of how closely young women were seen to adhere to these.

Such images and expected behaviour clash with the self-image of many working women, who have new styles of clothing and habits of consumption, a sense of independence and a willingness to justify their new ways of doing things. Many women say that complying with customary rules and expectations is simply unrealistic in a world where men can no longer provide for their children and support their families. As some of the respondents explained, they do not wish to disrespect tradition or undermine the older generation, but are simply being realistic about the challenges of post-apartheid poverty and the need to grasp opportunities that present themselves. Young working women argue that they are forced to "tighten the belt" in a situation where the patriarchs are failing them.[32]

Under lockdown, pressure was imposed on women to comply with more conservative household regimens and to display greater support for the family and less inclination towards independence. Men and older women have used the process of domestic confinement to re-assert power and authority in the household, calling younger women to order and placing them under pressure. Many of those interviewed said that more food was consumed when people were locked down because they were not busy outside the household sphere. This placed pressure on household finances because food prices had risen during lockdown. Men demanded that meals be prepared and that women put food on the table when they were hungry. A health official from one of the communities reported dealing with cases of injuries to the women who had been beaten by their husbands due to frustrations at an absence of food. The official stated:

> People's everyday routines are negatively affected because now people are not working but they used to work, and this affected poverty as well as food security and ultimately is leading to domestic violence. We have had patients who were beaten by their husbands because *akusekho mvisiswano kumama notata, utata nomama abanamali*, so the other one is blaming the other one, and this leads to domestic violence because there is no food.

In times of hunger and scarcity, women carry a heavy load because they are supposed to activate neighbourhood networks of sharing and the kinship relations that will ensure that resources continue to flow into the household for its survival. This is difficult to achieve when you are not able to move around, visit neighbours or travel to the cities and towns to engage the wives of close relatives and friends, or even to activate mutual support networks in the villages. Moreover, before lockdowns there was already a crisis of social reproduction in rural areas; many homesteads were hungry and desperate. The responsibility of protecting household members from even greater vulnerability has fallen disproportionately on women, but they cannot fulfil these duties under lockdown. Their families look to them for greater compliance and provision and labour to ensure social reproduction, which is seemingly impossible under the circumstances. As expectations are thwarted, domestic violence erupts as men turn on their wives and lovers for not activating their networks to put food on the table. Older men and women also feel the pressure and expect younger women to fill the gap and carry the load—to work harder in and for the household in the time of Covid-19. Women resist these attempts to shackle them because they have come to expect greater freedom and independence, and now feel hemmed in by the proximity of greater domestic control at home. Already fraught relationships and interpersonal violence within rural households have been exacerbated in many areas. The surge of such violence across the country led President Cyril Ramaphosa to declare that gender and domestic violence was a pandemic of equal magnitude to that of Covid-19.[33]

In this time of scarcity and lockdown, the gate was closing in rural communities across the former Transkei. This occurred at precisely the time of year that the gate would normally be opening with the social mobilisation of households and communities between Easter and harvesting, and the departure of the male youth to the mountains. Like Christmas, this is a time of greater sharing and solidarity in rural communities, between households that otherwise live in greater isolation and under constant stress to make ends meet. Massive outmigration has produced social thinning in rural areas and households. In many instances, the entire middle generation is no longer there because they have left for the cities. Those who remain behind find few work opportunities and depend heavily on welfare grants and state transfers for their survival. Some command of the English language is a basic requirement these days for virtually any form of employment in South Africa, and schools are notoriously poor in the rural areas, which means that such skills are difficult to acquire unless young people leave for the cities. But not everyone can go, and there are those who feel obliged to stay behind to help their mothers and grandparents with responsibilities at home. There is already a high level of isolation and vulnerability in rural areas today, where female-headed households are locked down in poverty in places from which they are unable to escape. In many rural areas there is also rising rural crime, much of which is perpetrated by unemployed male youths.

Collective action is often the only way to keep a lid on rural crime and stock theft. Historically, this has not been tackled by the police; instead senior men in the community have come together to galvanise an anti-crime drive and contain the problem. Community vigilantism has always been a key strategy against stock theft and petty crime in rural areas. Crime is contained when community members are communicating and able to stand together, track down criminals, and expose them. Conditions of social isolation and social distancing benefit criminals in rural areas because they can act with impunity. In this regard, even the chiefs said the conditions produced under Covid-19 and lockdown were a challenge.

Gender-based violence, witchcraft related crimes and Covid-19

In colonial Africa, there was a widespread belief that witchcraft would disappear as the continent embarked on new processes of social change. However, when urbanisation, modernisation and expanded Christianisation took people away from their rural homes and traditions, this disappearance never materialised. In fact, by the 1980s it was widely recognised that increased levels of insecurity and strain within both urban and rural communities actually escalated witchcraft related activity throughout Africa. It was widely recognised that witchcraft related beliefs and actions were not likely to fade with the arrival of modernity, as anthropologists had once predicted. Instead, they were part of everyday life in post-colonial Africa, and especially in the large cities from Johannesburg to Kinshasa and Lagos, where social, economic and spiritual insecurity prevailed.[34] Adam Ashworth wrote that in South Africa after apartheid, there were many more cases of witchcraft accusation and witchcraft related crimes in Soweto and the townships of Johannesburg than in the countryside. This was because of rising levels of economic and especially *spiritual* insecurity, associated with job losses, political change, ethnic mixing and the arrival of African nationals from all over the continent.[35]

However, there are also studies which demonstrate that witchcraft accusations and witchcraft related crimes were on the increase in rural areas as well, especially where ANC comrades and elders had been struggling for power. The work of Isak Niehaus in the former Lebowa homeland shows that the transition to democracy brokered a sharp increase in witchcraft related violence and activities in this area.[36] He traced this back to the 1960s, when chiefs and traditional leaders lost legitimacy in the homeland after they were co-opted by the apartheid state. However, the steady growth of cases exploded into widespread witchcraft related activity when local leaders openly challenged the power of chiefs and tribal authorities as they struggled for power. Political adversaries were named as evil agents, and were often stigmatised as witches, or the agents of witches. Witchcraft activity was also seen in accusations of villagers being murdered for the use of their body parts or *muti*. Similar outbreak of witchcraft related killings and accusations occurred in other former homelands, such as Venda and especially KwaZulu-Natal,[37] which was engulfed in factional political violence throughout the 1990s.[38] In the former Transkei, there was little violence and instability associated with the transition from apartheid to the new post-apartheid dispensation. The period of relative stability can be contrasted to the volatile 1950s, when the Bantu Authorities Act of 1951 was being implemented in the region and there was constant upheaval and violence, some of which was witchcraft related.[39] In the period after 2000, and espe-cially into the 2010s, when so much social change and death gripped the countryside, there was a resurgence of witchcraft related crimes and violence. This is confirmed in the work of Eastern Cape anthro-pologist, Theodor Petrus, who confirms that Pondoland has histori-cally been a regional hotspot for witchcraft related crimes, as the north-eastern part of the region generally has registered the largest number of cases. While doing research in the Transkei in the 2000s, he noted that official cases reported were the tip of the iceberg of witchcraft related crime in this region.[40]

In the 2000s, Petrus noted that the impact of HIV and AIDS on rural communities contributed to the rising witchcraft cases because the pandemic particularly affected the youth. As these deaths were unnatural, they generated spiritual insecurity and uncertainty in rural homes and communities. In one case, an older women was accused of being a witch, and confessed to killing many young men and women in the village. She said that she had infected them with HIV and AIDS through a witchcraft technique called *ukuthgwebula*, where the witch magically extracted fluids from one body and inserted them in another, thus spreading the infection at will. In this case, Petrus says that the woman warned the community that the infected youth would not live out the year. When this came to pass, she was hunted down and killed. The sudden death of young people—possible future breadwinners—caused communities to seek out witches, whom they believed have the power of *ukuthqwebula*. They also targeted traditional healers, who they thought were being manipulated by witches to produce dangerous and invisible ways of spreading HIV and AIDS.[41] Petrus also notes that, while the police normally pursue anyone responsible for murder and gender-based violence (GBV), in some cases the community believes that the witchcraft allegations are valid and that the "witches" should be punished. They agree with the witch naming and support the pursuit of certain women as witches. Petrus sees this as a problem for the police since it is not a crime to behave like a witch, whereas those who attack or assault alleged witches, on the other hand, are immediately liable for arrest and prosecution. Petrus suggests that the law should recognise that witchcraft is a real and present threat in rural communities, which believe in the existence of supernatural forces and the capacities of witches to destroy lives and property.[42]

In a 2012 essay, Petrus explores the political and economic context of the rise in witchcraft related crime in the Eastern Cape after 2000. He argues that conditions of poverty and inequality exacerbate the possibility for witchcraft. He also notes, alongside others like Niehaus,[43] that because traditional leaders are also state bureaucrats, they have remained alienated from their former roles as leaders who commanded spiritual powers and engaged with supernatural forces.[44] When these forces are not controlled by chiefs, they can fall into the hands of others, including corrupt traditional healers, who do not always have the best interests of the community at heart. Covid, and the fear and suspicion it created, has increased the incidence of witchcraft accusations and violence in the Eastern Cape. In fact, funerals often provided the catalytic moments that resulted in the activation of witch-hunts, led by young men who are often inspired by the presence of urban youth. In March 2020, a group of youths who attended the funeral of a young man in Majuba village in Sterkspruit in the former Transkei descended on the home of an 83-year-old widow, Nosayinethi Manundu. They alleged that a young man's death in the location was caused by the action of this woman, who was a witch. The final decision to attack and kill the old widow was taken after the funeral on the Saturday, where youths grappled with the unnatural death of a peer. The woman was murdered 24 hours after the funeral finished. The attack was not the act of a single person, but of a group of young men, four of whom were arrested by the local police. One escaped to Western Cape, where he was found stabbed to death the week after the incident. The witchcraft related violence left the family of the deceased and the community traumatised, as many feared that there might be more killings in the area. The mob who attached Nosayinethi Manundu poured paraffin on her 23-year-old granddaughter, but the liquid did not ignite. A 38-year-old relative of the deceased women said that she feared for her life because the "old women died like a dog", and those who murdered her could "come for others". The granddaughter said that: "after the incident, we no longer trust anyone here, as we have been getting threatening calls. I am struggling to sleep at night as I can still hear my grandmother screaming and begging for her life".

In July 2020, a group of young men accused four women of being witches in the Embihli village in Senqu Municipality. They shot and killed three of the women and critically injured the fourth. The incident seemed to follow the same pattern of previous cases. The women were accused of causing harm and death to youths in the village by working together. The mayor of the Senqu Municiaplity, Nomvuyo Mposelwa confirmed that the violence was once again the work of young men, who are "not stopping this Gender Based Violence".[45] She said that the incident was a tragedy, especially since it occurred: "as we enter August, Women's Month, a number of these cases are being reported. It is time for all women in the country to say in one voice, women's lives matter".[46] In another case recorded in September 2020, a group of vigilantes in the Transkei managed to track down three young men, who were alleged to have murdered a female witch. The community vigilantes beat the men before they were handed over to the police. In other cases, however, when the community supported the youths' allegations of witchcraft, they would protect them from prosecution and hide their identities from the police.

In another series of cases, it was reported that villagers close to the birthplace of the late ANC struggle icon Winnie Madikizela-Mandela were living in fear, after more than 33 people had been murdered in in Bizana district of Pondoland. Of those murdered, 16 were women, who were hacked to death after being accused of witchcraft. One victim, a 78-year-old woman called Ntombizodwa Toto Madikileza was murdered by assailants in the middle of the night in front of her 13 grandchildren. Connie Madikizela said that: "so many children have been orphaned in the wave of witch killings because our old women look after and foster many children here".[47] She said that the whole community felt terrorised by "gangs of young men moving around with axes alleging they had identified witches, whom they wanted to kill". The local headman Inkosi Nobomi Madikizela said that attacks were out of hand in the area, and he did not know how to contain the cycle of violence and counter-violence that had gripped the Bizana area. In her review of violence and witchcraft in rural communities in the 1940s and 1950s, Sean Reading emphasises that these accusations and witchcraft related crime were often confined to families; this appears to be the case in the Madikizela family or clan in Bizana.

However, witchcraft accusations and vigilante activities seem to have become intertwined. The surge of witchcraft accusations and killing in the locations appears connected to the growth of visible inequalities in the built environment of rural areas, which are rapidly changing and modernising as increasing numbers of people spend most of their time in the cities. At the end of apartheid, village land-scapes in the Transkei looked remarkably uniform and egalitarian, dominating by traditional blue, white and grey, wattle and daub *rondwels*, which were almost identical in size, shape and spatial orien-tation. The transformation of built environment across the Transkei has produced marked social differentiation. Equivalence amongst kin and neighbours has dissolved into growing competition and envy.

If the escalation of witchcraft related crime and violence in the rural Transkei today is compared to previous decades, it appears that intra-community strife and violence have become much more signifi-cant than inter-community conflict. In the apartheid era, land was scarce and different ethnic communities or factions had to compete for limited resources. With a migrant labour system, the primary conflicts were horizontal, between locations or sections of locations. This was expressed primarily through faction fights or neighbourhood conflicts, where male youth from one village section or mine hostel would battle with those from other sections or hostels. The conflicts were underpinned by male solidarity and a politics of ethnic or resi-dential equivalence. These factional disputes over land and territory are no longer so evident in the Transkei, where agrarianism is less important to rural livelihoods than in the heyday of apartheid. The conflicts and competition between families is now significant. Competition entrenches itself on the rural landscape through the look and style of suburban homes and access to the trappings of a consumer lifestyle. In this context of growing poverty, desperation and material inequality, the idiom, imagination, and practice of witchcraft has re-emerged as an increasingly common feature of everyday village life. The primary victims of this violence are old women. Youths believe that, after decades of grappling with the AIDS pandemic, they are using their power to destroy the lives of young men and women, whom they resent for leaving the locations for the cities. Indeed, as Sean Reading notes, elderly rural women are targeted as witches not because they are weak and powerless, but rather because they are believed to have considerable generational and spiritual power, which they can use to destroy the lives of others. Young men, in both the rural and urban areas, seem to regard their misfortunes and thwarted masculinities as the work of powerful rural women.

Conclusion

We began this chapter with a discussion of reverse migration in India at the start of lockdown, when livelihood options in cities disappeared and the global media captured human trains of returning migrants walking home, across hundreds or even thousands of miles. Many of these migrants moved annually between family farms in the country-side and urban opportunities in the city. In South Africa, the involve-

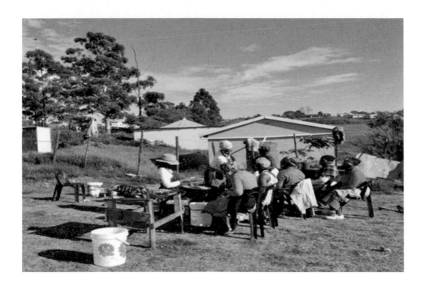

Fig. 1: Women prepare food for a rural funeral in Mhlanga village, Oliver Tambo District, April 2020 (photo: Phindile Siyasanga Shinga)

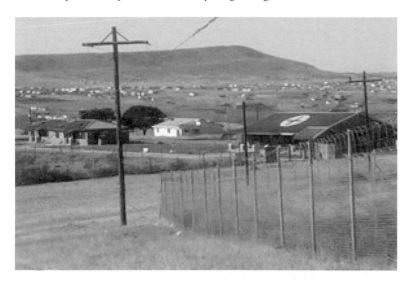

Fig. 2: Many rural clinics, police stations and government offices were closed at the peak of infections due to a lack of protective equipment, June 2020 (photo: Bukeka Shumane)

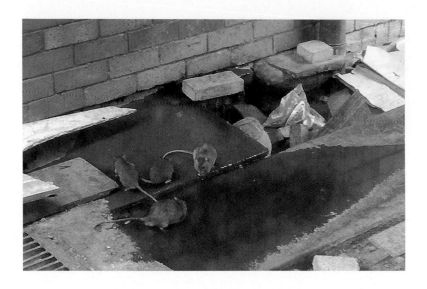

Fig. 3: Rats licking blood from the drains at Livingstone Hospital, July 2020 (photo: Estelle Ellis)

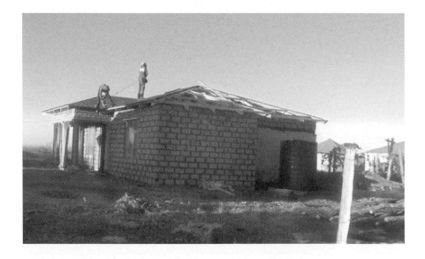

Fig. 4: Modernising rural homesteads in the rural Eastern Cape (photo: Sanele Krishe)

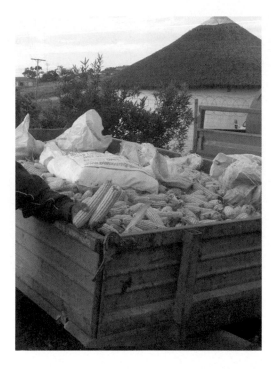

Figs 5a, b: Homestead harvest scenes, May 2020 (photos: Athi Phiwani)

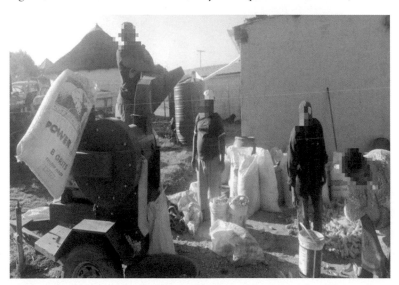

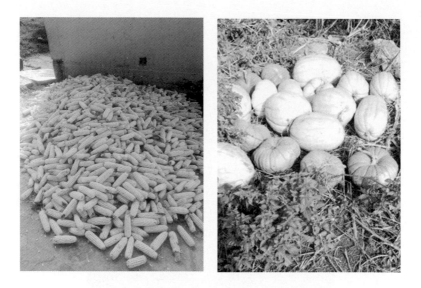

Figs 5 c, d: Homestead harvest scenes, May 2020 (photos: Athi Phiwani)

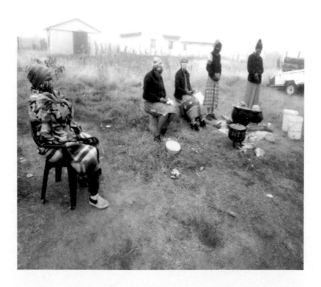

Fig. 6: Women attempt to keep their distance as they prepare food outside for a funeral (photo: Mandlakazi Tshunungwa)

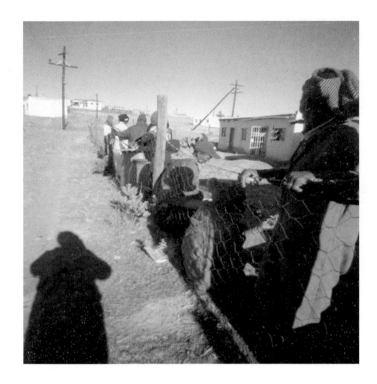

Figs 7 (*above*), 8 (*below*): Keeping behind the garden gate in Nqwala village (photo: Puleng Moruri), while dense crowds gather as bottle stores reopen in Bizana town in OR Tambo district in the former Transkei (photo: Phindile Siyasanga Shinga)

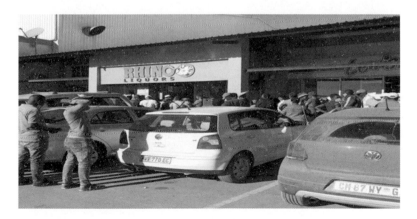

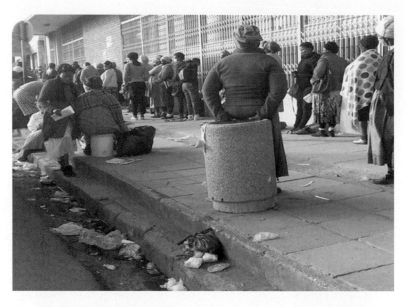

Fig. 9: Long queues for social grants at the Mthatha town post office, 7 July 2020 (photo: Nelly Sharpley)

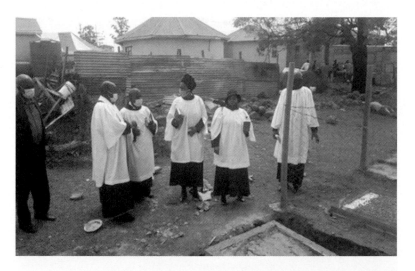

Fig. 10: Pastoral presence of church leaders at the grave side, many infected (photo: Bukeka Shumane)

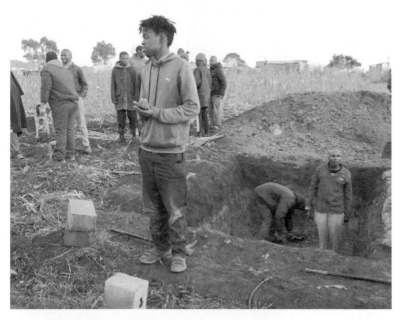

Fig. 11: Gravediggers at work behind the homestead maize field in Bizana (photo: Phindile Siyasanga Shinga)

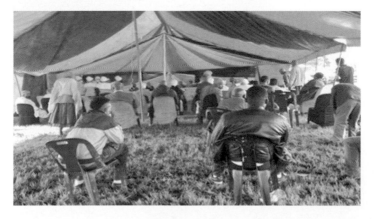

Fig. 12: Dwindling numbers at rural funerals in the second wave in Bizana (photo: Zipho Xego)

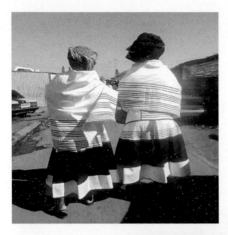

Fig. 13: Women dress in traditional clothes for a reburial in Bizana (photo: Zipho Xego)

Fig. 14: Relatives and village youths bring blanketed initiates back from the hills to the village in Bizana, January 2021 (photo: Phindile Siyasanga Shinga)

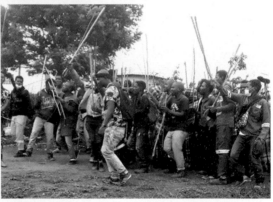

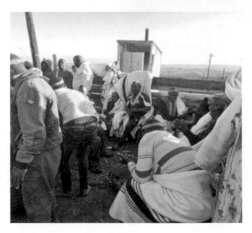

Fig. 15: Cape Town migrant (*seated centre*) returns home for a ritual to honour the ancestors and his father, September 2021 (photo: Sanele Krishe)

ment of migrants in interconnected livelihood pursuits between town and country is less pronounced, especially since government grants are available in rural areas and families rely less on farming and cash remittance for survival than in the past. However, as we have argued above, this has not reduced double-rootedness; urbanising families continue to invest in their rural homestead in various ways and frequently return home for family rituals and retirement. Between March and June 2020, 15% of South African households changed shape with new arrivals or departures in the face of the Covid crisis. A considerable number of those who moved went home, especially over the Easter period, and did not return to the cities after the lockdown window shut. In the rural areas, homestead gates were also shut when the lockdown set in and people feared arrest if they were caught in the streets, travelling to town or visiting neighbours or friends.

The chapter has explored the efforts of the elderly in households to encourage social cohesion and common purpose. Youth and women were now accustomed to independence and freedom outside of the moral constraints of older social hierarchies and obligations. We have explored how this created tension "behind the garden gate", especially since the elders regarded the desire of the younger generation to move around as threatening to their health. Movement was, however, often necessitated by a desire to find income and opportunity, rather than to deliberately defy the law or disobey the wishes of matriarchs or patriarchs at home. Special pressure was placed on women to use their networks to activate sharing and inter-household exchange. The chapter explores these dynamics in the historical context of labour migration, and the recent absence of co-operative labour and close neighbourly relations in rural areas. In fact, as Ngwane explained, the idea of tight household cohesion was more a script of hope than an everyday reality in rural areas. As youth, women and elders all saw their rural homes as valued places to dwell, visit, build and belong, there was intensified gender and generational conflict during lockdown, resulting in the South African President calling GBV a parallel pandemic to Covid-19.

The final part of the chapter explored how these struggles were not new. They have been playing themselves out for some time through the connections between ritual events such as funerals, when urban migrants return to the countryside, and conflicts over access to power and rural resources, as expressed in witchcraft accusations. The chapter highlights the way in which Covid has enlivened some of these ongoing struggles, expressed through idioms of custom. This theme will be explored in more detail in chapter six, where we discuss the return to customary practices as the second wave of infections passed through the countryside at the end of 2020.

5

GATEKEEPERS

Introduction

Customary practices in rural areas are fluid and changing. As one respondent noted: "there is no bible documenting our traditions where you can point to the passages and the verses of what needs to be done, or which way is the right way".[1] He said that, "Ours is an oral tradition, it depends on the knowledge old people have of how our customs are meant to be performed, but also what passes as the correct or adequate way of doing things is always open to persuasion and change". In the rural villages of the Eastern Cape in 2020, customary practices are far from homogenous or monolithic. They are dynamic and often differ from one area or family to the next, as different versions of custom have been adopted and performed. Families, individuals, churches, healers and even state officials can influence the way things are done. However, within this diversity and contestation, the key concern is always whether the ritual can do the cultural work for which it is intended. Can it secure a legitimate passage from boyhood to manhood, make a woman a respected wife, or carry the spirit of a deceased man or woman from this life to the next? Today, as is always the case in times of crisis, the shape and meaning of ritual and custom is still in constant dispute, between gender and generations, between the old and the new, between different families and clans.

But local people say that cutting corners or making radical changes in ritual practices can be dangerous and lead to spiritual anxiety and family misfortune. If villagers cut the time allocated to rituals, miss out phases, ignore critical elements in the sequence or fail to cook and distribute food and drink in a customary manner, they might face consequences in the future. This view applies as much to funerals as it does to initiation rites or any other rite of passage.

The involvement of the state in customary affairs has already been well-established in the Eastern Cape, with the constant debate around male initiation and public health and safety. The level and nature of the state's involvement is nevertheless limited here to protect the cultural legitimacy of the rite of passage. The distribution of a documentary called *Inxeba* (the wound) created a stir in South Africa in 2019. It detailed the experience of a gay youth in an initiation lodge and included secret footage of youths in seclusion in the bush in the Eastern Cape. Xhosa heterosexual men and cultural groups mobilised to have the documentary banned on the grounds that it undermined their cultural rights and the legitimacy of Xhosa male initiation by making their cultural secrets public.[2] The issue of secrecy and ritual is also dealt with in Jonathan Stadler's book *Public Secrets and Private Sufferings in the South African AIDS Epidemic*. He explores how families and individuals remain silent on the causes of their illnesses and perform rituals where the real reasons for death in the family members are never disclosed. He shows how funerals have become ritual space where the family business is done in public to protect private secrets and limit the extent of external intervention and state control in family matters.[3]

In 2020 the state created a special state of exception, where rites of passage were suspended in rural areas and rural funerals were radically restructured. Families were unnerved and confused. As the regulations became tighter and increasingly invasive and controlling, the integrity and power of custom appeared to be compromised. In his 2016 book, *Ebola: How People's Science Helped End an Epidemic*, Paul Richards showed how the World Health Organization (WHO) and other international agencies realised the benefits of focusing on community engagement and home-care, instead of radical isolation and containment, in their approach to management of Ebola outbreaks.[4]

After initially trying to remove people who were at risk of infection or already infected for specialised treatment and containment in field hospital facilities, the WHO and others were eventually persuaded that more could be achieved by working collaboratively with traditional leaders, burial societies and ordinary people. Médecins Sans Frontières (MSF) took the lead in calling on international agencies to focus more on therapeutic care than containment.[5] With death occurring in 50 to 90 percent of cases and medical proof that bodies of Ebola victims remained highly infections after death, there was much emphasis on the nature of funerals. The immediate inclination of the WHO and the international bio-medical teams was to get the bodies wrapped in plastic and buried as soon as possible. But burying bodies without appropriate rituals and approval by secret burial societies could mean that the spirit of the deceased and the families left behind could be cursed.[6] The issue came to a head when a local WHO team pushed to rapidly bury a body of a pregnant young woman far away from the village, but locals were determined to do funeral rites in a customary fashion and remove the foetus to avoid a curse on the family. This decision was reversed though the involvement of an intermediatory as the WHO team agreed to meet the community and eventually paid for a customary funeral, where the foetus was removed and customary practices instituted with due care and caution.[7]

With the outbreak of Covid in South Africa, the state never advocated radical measures for the disposal of bodies far away from villages, homes and communities, although the President did encourage people to stay away from funerals, which were governed by tight restrictions. During the first wave in 2020, the President's advisory council was comprised entirely of bio-medical experts. There were no anthropologists, social scientists or community members offering mitigating perspectives like those presented by anthropologists and community leaders in the West African Ebola debate. The state was in charge and determined to enforce its top-down prescriptions, leaving little room for flexibility, local voices, cultural compromises and care. This changed to some degree with the inclusion of social scientists in the Command Council and the decision in January 2021 to remove the compulsory burial of bodies in plastic. In 2020, however, the President appealed to communities to leave their customs aside until the virus was under control. In the rural locations, this was not an option, especially since death was ever present and escalating daily. The South African state and medical establishment boxed custom into a corner and used the familiar discourse of custom as "super spreader" to deflect attention from the limitations of its own polices. In doing this, the gate was closed, *ukuvala isango*, on rural communities, who were left to negotiate culturally legitimate and meaningful rites of passage under adverse conditions. The focus of this chapter is on the different stakeholders involved, especially the gatekeepers and brokers at the local level. The chapter explores their attitudes, roles and orientations in the Covid crisis as they were involved in managing death and distress in rural communities from April to July 2020. The chapter shows that local elites and gatekeepers were often on the side of the state rather than the people, as they helped enforce immediate lockdown and rural compliance.

Fear, compliance and leadership

Traditional and religious leaders and ward councillors reported significant levels of fear of the Covid-19 virus across the region. Local people were reportedly aware that "thousands" were dying of the virus; that it was airborne; and that it had no cure—"this virus kills even nurses and doctors". People were particularly frightened by the speed with which the virus could kill people and because they could not tell who was infected. They compared the uncertainty over the threat posed by Covid-19 with their relative clarity on the causes, symptoms and treatment for HIV and AIDS—"with Covid-19, you never know". Seen by some initially as a white person's disease, a significant number of leaders expressed the popular view that travel and tourism were to blame for its early spread in the Eastern Cape—in particular during the few days of May when official inter-provincial restrictions on movement were lifted. Several leaders reported the view that funerals had contributed to the spread, with one traditional leader also blaming churches and a religious leader linking the lifting of travel restrictions and the holding of funerals as a cause—"people coming from the Western Cape attending the funerals brought this Coronavirus".

Views varied quite widely on the extent to which rural people were adhering to the government's rules on masks and social distancing. In general, the ward councillors were more likely to claim that their constituents were adhering to the rules; one claimed that "people even wear masks when they return from herding the cows". However, the consensus view among the leaders was more nuanced. People often wore masks when they went into town rather than in their villages. In part, this was because in the villages "they are in their comfortable spaces with people they know and trust—they don't practise social distancing when they fetch water from the well or visit friends". Leaders linked this inconsistent behaviour to higher levels of enforcement by police and other officials in urban areas, indicating a general lack of voluntary compliance. It was noted that people tended to talk about the rules rather than observe them, although the elderly and women clearly took the virus and the measures to prevent its spread more seriously than the youth.

In general, the leadership groups reported widespread popular cynicism in relation to the perceived value and impacts of the government's rules. Community leaders were particularly forthright on this point, noting that many local people did not seem that concerned by the outbreak and had continued their daily routines as usual without wearing masks or observing physical distancing. Popular cynicism was also noted in relation to drinking. Almost all the leaders reported concern that widespread alcohol consumption had undermined the purpose and effectiveness of efforts to restrict the spread of virus. People failed to physically distance when they drank, sharing bottles and, inadvertently, masks. It was also reported that drinkers had claimed that only those who didn't drink caught the virus.

A further challenge was raised about physical distancing in overcrowded queues to collect grants in town, despite the presence of queue marshalls. They also reported difficulties in collecting grants, particularly for the elderly. Ensuring adequate water supplies was a particularly pressing concern for traditional leaders and councillors, for whom this represented a key part of their mandate. Great concern was expressed around livelihoods under Covid-19—leaders widely agreed that there had been too few food parcels, and alleged favouritism in their distribution. Hunger, particularly among the elderly, and nutrition were also raised as key issues. In this regard, subsistence agriculture was seen as crucial; one community leader advised that "people should start growing their own food to avoid travelling to town". Meanwhile, there was broad consensus that under-equipped, inadequately staffed, poorly resourced and distant clinics, many of which had closed, were unable to respond properly to the local health needs created by the virus. Another repeated concern was the absence of any form of testing for Covid-19 for rural residents—other than that offered by prohibitively expensive providers in town.

Many among the leadership groups believed that the imposition of the government restrictions on gatherings, preventing people from coming together, had both undermined their own work and communal resilience more broadly. One traditional leader pointed out that without meetings, there was no work for him. A ward councillor noted that the committees, which were essential to his job, could no longer convene. Religious leaders described churches being closed and services being conducted via social media with congregants wearing masks. Community meetings were prohibited and contacts among villagers were hedged by fear, which only exacerbated the isolation of households within communities that were already fractured by anxiety over the outbreak. The breakdown of communal life was vividly described by one traditional leader, who noted that people no longer visited their neighbours as much because "everyone is afraid of death ... The only place people meet are funerals ... and then only because they don't have a choice". One religious leader said that Covid-19 had broken the "family bond of the congregation". He said people now feared the virus more than God, and were living unfamiliar, distant and anti-social lives.

At the same time, however, many of the local leaders supported the government's response to the virus. One traditional leader noted that "there would have been many people who would have been dead by now [in the absence of the official measures]". Another stressed the importance of adhering to the rules: "respect law as it [the virus] kills". A religious leader described the outcome of a meeting held by the South African Council of Churches (SACC): "We are not going to compromise, but comply with regulations." A common view was that greater police and even military visibility was required to ensure that a recalcitrant rural population was kept in line. Various members of the religious, traditional and political leadership groups described a role for themselves in this enforcement, particularly in relation to how funerals should be held. Some leaders felt that the state's increased engagement in everyday behaviours and practices had bolstered their local roles. One councillor said the virus had brought him closer to the community he served. For others, particularly the local community leaders, the rules and their enforcement were viewed as forms of state power that needed to be made more responsive to local needs.

Contestation over funerals

Views about the rules governing funerals, and local adherence to these, varied widely among the leadership groups. A significant number of traditional and religious leaders noted that the rules were largely being followed. However, councillors and community leaders tended to focus more on how they were breached, with many councillors emphasising community "disobedience". Community leaders focused more on how effective (or ineffective) the rules actually were: "[the government] interventions are working but not working". In large part, the differences in perspective may be related to the functions of the various leadership groups. At one end of the spectrum, the councillors and traditional leaders appeared to be seeking compliance with the state regulation of deaths and funerals. To do this they appointment local headmen to encourage compliance; ensured registration of deaths; engaged the various government enforcement, health and welfare agencies around preparations for funerals; provided sanitiser and registers; and monitored compliance with the rules at these events. The religious leaders, by contrast, seemed to be trying to combine their pastoral and religious duties with efforts to make sure that the rules were being followed, particularly in terms of the order of service and length of the funerals. They left compliance over other issues, such as counting the numbers of attendees, to other actors like the councillors and the police. Meanwhile, the priority of community leaders was not always to ensure observance of the regulations; one stated the regulations were popularly perceived as "ridiculous". Instead, community leaders appeared to focus more on adapting community behaviours to the new regulatory dispensation, while interrogating the effectiveness and appropriateness of the rules against the yardstick of customary social and cultural behaviour.

Notwithstanding their differences of perspecti ·es, a number of common views emerged among the leadership stakehoiders. It was widely felt that the restrictions on the duration of the whole funeral process, including the actual funeral service and burial ceremony, and on the number of attendees, were of significant benefit to poorer families. The shorter, smaller funerals saved them a great deal of unnecessary expense, described by one respondent as "waste", and, to an extent, created more democratic funeral practices. One traditional leader decried lavish burials, which were viewed as a relatively recent phenomenon, as a form of "Western" materialism—"funerals like weddings". All leadership groups also saw shorter funerals as saving valuable time—although this was mainly from the point of view of their own convenience, freeing them to attend to other business. As one councillor said: "The old programme was just wasting time".

The stakeholders were also almost unanimous in describing the cultural harm caused by new rules on the handling of Covid-19 corpses and how these were being implemented. In particular, they criticised the ways in which family members were being prevented from viewing the corpses of loved ones. As one ward councillor said: "Culturally, the whole community is bleeding." The rules were seen to prevent families from communicating with the spirits of the recently departed; they were not able to ward off the threat that they could pose to the living. The possibility of burying the wrong body—which was widely reported to have happened in several cases across the Eastern Cape—was viewed as the ultimate wrong that could be inflicted by adherence to this rule. Thus, the restrictions were seen not only as a cause of great fear and anguish, but also as prompting dramatic acts of defiance—such as when relatives forced open coffins before burial in order to identify the body and communicate with them one last time, out of fear of being haunted. In one case, according to one religious leader, a coffin was pried open during the funeral cortege because it looked too short to accommodate the corpse—a supposition that proved correct.

There was unanimity among the stakeholders about the depth and scale of the distress caused by the restrictions on access to the body. However, views diverged on the precise nature and consequences of family and community responses to the restrictions, as well as how to address this distress. Again, the divergence in views among the leadership groups may, to an extent, be attributed to their perceptions of their own roles in the process. For example, several councillors described grief-stricken, fearful family members' efforts to force open coffins as a form of defiance or disobedience—"people treat the rules as a joke"—which caused further infection: "the one that forced and opened their sister's coffin, now they are all sick in the household, and probably with Covid-19". For these councillors, people's happiness with the restrictions was irrelevant: "they just have to be comfortable with the laws". If the rules were not followed, reports of disobedience were passed by councillors and their proxies to the police to force compliance. As once councillor complained, this sometimes created "unnecessary enemies" in the community.

An interesting theme in the councillors' accounts was a tendency to simultaneously proclaim that the rules were being variously "warmed to", "respected" and followed "without hesitation"—"people accept wrapping as a good regulation"—while also acknowledging that these rules were being flouted. One councillor noted that he was duty-bound to keep a record of all deaths and their causes, and said that people were no longer informing the office "especially if the death is Covid-19 related". He claimed that "when you visit the unreported funerals you will find that none of the regulations are followed". This narrative strategy portrays those who break the rules as aberrant—"not all families have been honest"—and also identifies them as a cause of infection, particularly since many councillors maintained that funerals themselves were inherently dangerous. Another councillor claimed that "after funerals, there are always many people who are infected without being sure where they got it from". Similarly, one traditional leader feared the spread of the disease from the dead bodies themselves, if people persisted in breaking the rules for handling them.

In this climate of fear, a number of respondents felt that the rules on death and funerals, and their implementation, seemed predicated on the view that all current deaths could be attributed to Covid-19. As one community leader noted, the rule that only the family could attend funerals assumed that people were hiding the cause of death when it was Covid-19. Another community leader wondered: "why do funeral parlours treat every body as if it were a Covid-19 case?" This interrogation of the purpose and usefulness of the regulations on handling bodies, and the impact of these regulations on the usual ways of addressing and burying the dead, was expanded on by a number of the traditional and community leaders and one of the councillors. They sought to distinguish between the customs around preparing bodies for burial and the cultural significance attached to these customs; and were open to the possibility of finding new ways of managing death and bereavement that satisfied cultural demands while also protecting the living from the outbreak. For example, one traditional leader supported the relative simplicity and speed of burials under Covid-19, referencing older burial practices: "this is how funerals used to be held, on the day or soon after death, with the body taken to the graveyard wrapped in a cloth (*ingcawe*) or dress (*umbhaco*)." Another advocated the reintroduction of the practice of so-called secret burials, or *ukuqhusheka*, under which it is permissible to bury someone quickly and without great ceremony. This senior traditional leader indicated that such burials were practical, saved poor families money and met the needs of ancestors who understood that current conditions precluded long ceremonies.

The difference between modern and traditional funeral customs was amplified in another comment by a traditional leader who described the rites of gravedigging prevalent at many burials as a "custom, not a cultural practice". As gravedigging times were cut under the new Covid-19 dispensation, one community leader described how a village started using mechanical diggers. At the same time, some rituals have quietly persisted. These include the brewing of beer to cleanse the gravedigging spades and the ritual slaughter of animals, although sheep were often used rather than cows, which are deemed too much of a "crowd-puller", in one community leader's words. The need to adjust culture as a "way of protecting the ones who are still alive" was particularly addressed by community leaders, although also by other leadership groups, in different ways. It was seen as a source of some difficulty, particularly by the priests, who were sympathetic to the plight of families unable to view their loved ones but emphasised that the rules should be followed. As one said: "There is nothing that can be done because the government has spoken." The leaders who adopted this kind of stance proposed few immediate solutions, instead kicking the can down the road. One pastor mentioned that church ceremonies "raising the jackets" of dead congregants in their honour had been postponed due to the danger posed by large assemblies. Traditional leaders expressed concern that local people who had died in other provinces would be buried there and not at their home spaces. One spoke of the need "to conduct certain rituals to right the wrongs necessitated by Coronavirus in accordance with our traditions". A religious leader spoke of the prospect of many reburials after the outbreak had passed, with another indicating that at least one reburial had already taken place after the spirit of a late father had complained.

In terms of seeking some compromise between the rules and cultural practices, leaders across all groups recommended allowing families to at least see the face of the deceased; they agreed that funeral parlours should wrap the bodies so that the face would be visible. One traditional leader proposed relaxing the rules on numbers at funerals, suggesting that instead he and his peers should ensure physical distancing at these events. Generally, it was community and traditional leaders who particularly interrogated the validity of the rules and came up with broader proposals for action to change them. One traditional leader proposed a workshop on the issue of wrapping bodies in plastic, which was considered by many of the leaders as antithetical to Xhosa cultural treatment of the dead, in which the flesh must meet the soil. Other traditional leaders linked their discontent with some of the rules to a broader lack of engagement by the national government with chiefs; they felt that the chiefs were under-represented in official political structures.

For community leaders, a greater priority seemed to have been incorporating some meaning into burials during the outbreak. As one councillor noted: "Even the ancestors know the crisis of Covid-19", indicating that paths to alternative ways of appeasing the recently deceased may be found, in coordination with their spirits. The focus was mainly on how the body is handled and moved—and the viewing and talking that should accompany this—rather than on the funeral itself. The bodies of the dead are seen by the families of the deceased as "theirs". Their passage from life to death must be handled with great care. One community leader said:

> We are worried ancestors will turn their backs on us if we throw our people into the ground without even viewing the body. The body should be viewed at the parlour before loading onto the hearse and once again when it arrives home. We must be given time to talk to it the way we want. Families must be able to explain to the deceased what is happening.

A Methodist preacher confirmed that they had been instructed by their church elders to allow the family to see the body in leaving the parlour and when arriving at their home "to check it is the right one and for closure". He said that if the body was not seen, it "made an unbearable scar because it is painful not to see your loved one for the last time. … People are being buried as if they are stillborn babies, which is improper." Another religious leader said, "people still need to live despite the pandemic and their living include worshipping their ancestors."

In seeking to adapt the rules to fit people's psychological and emotional needs, one community leader noted: "People should opt for cultural evolution—understanding that some rituals will change although their meaning doesn't." Local scholar and cultural specialist Professor Somadoda Fikeni noted that traditional practices, such as those for funerals, had been subject to negotiated settlement for many years—varying among the various belief systems of family members and in response to material conditions. Fikeni stressed the cultural importance of observing the wishes of the dead; bringing the body back home; producing rites appropriate to the social status of the deceased; and ensuring that the necessary rituals were conducted to protect the body from witchcraft. Fikeni said that negotiations to alter customs should seek to provide a bridge from the known to the new and thus had to be conducted in close collaboration with the people. At one community meeting, it was decided that people would be buried according to custom. An official complaint was lodged by one community about the need for families to identify the body. Questions were also raised about the present practice of the bodies now being dressed by the morticians at the funeral parlour, and not by the family. In addition, given that the regulations governing funerals were, at best, being observed haphazardly, one community opted to elect a representative to coordinate with the police who were viewed as ineffective and not taken seriously locally.

Changing roles and responsibilities

Most of the leaders in the various groups indicated that the outbreak and lockdown rules had changed and sometimes restricted their roles within the community, particularly in relation to funerals. In part, their roles had become more limited as a result of fears for their own health and the risk of spreading the virus themselves. Traditional leaders described their continuing role in helping families to source death certificates, but said that they were no longer required to address mourners at funerals. These leaders also described new responsibilities in ensuring compliance with the rules on physical distancing, mask-wearing and sanitising at funerals, including ensuring that the municipality provided enough sanitiser for these events. They also made sure that tents were no longer erected for funeral parties and that numbers were checked. In some cases, these leaders delegated responsibility for attending funerals as representatives of the Great Place to one of their subjects, particularly if the event was not nearby. Religious leaders described post-lockdown funeral rites as isolated affairs—"generally, families are left alone to comfort and console themselves"—and noted that many local people had objected to the ban on overnight vigils on the eve of the funeral. They further noted a significant number of instances in which the restrictions on attendance numbers had been flouted, describing the attendance registers as "ineffective". One leader described how people were holding funerals "very early" so that they could be completed before the officials arrived, thus relieving the family of the responsibility of adhering to attendance limits by chasing people away, which they were unwilling to do.

Religious leaders described their pastoral role, advising parishioners on the impacts of the pandemic and the behavioural changes required to stop its spread, and supporting the bereaved with home visits, although one leader reported that these had been curtailed. They also described their roles in planning funerals in coordination with bereaved families to ensure that the rules were followed: "it is depressing because it is like we work hand in hand with the Department of Health—but our immediate priority is to save lives." They tried to ensure that funerals were short—with some aiming for ceremonies of less than one hour and others allowing up to two hours. They also noted that the length of their sermons had been cut, although at least the congregation was "not as tired" when these were delivered. However, several religious leaders were unwilling to take responsibility for the numbers attending funerals. One noted that local people regarded the rules restricting numbers as discriminatory. Another said it was for the councillors and the police to count the number of attendees. Preachers described the threat of infection that they faced in their pastoral work: "I feel like not attending funerals, but I cannot abandon church members".

Councillors described their role as essentially coordinating to ensure that bereaved families were made aware of the rules around funerals and complied with them. They deployed health workers, police and environmental affairs officials to instruct people how to prepare for funerals and then attended funerals in person, virtually or by proxy to ensure compliance. One councillor described visiting families to explain the guidelines, including the use of attendance registers for contact-tracing purposes (which was the only reference to this function of the registers among the respondents). Councillors described handing out sanitiser and registers. They also said that they were charged with keeping records of deaths, including causes of deaths, in their constituencies and reporting these to the municipality, as well as arranging follow-up screening of family members for cases of Covid-19 deaths. However, they noted that it was not always possible to ascertain the cause of death before burial. Community leaders primarily described their roles as supporting families in the practicalities of preparing for funerals, such as coordinating youth to help prepare food for attendees or even dig graves. However, they reported disruption to community life as a whole—"during this time not a single community meeting has been held, people are just doing what they think is right for them"—and to the activities associated with funerals, with many fewer supportive home visits being conducted. As one said: "Now only a few people go the day before to give money." Similarly, burial societies were reported to have closed and changed their constitutions, now contributing money instead of food. This change in the form of support offered to grieving families produced wider impacts in villages, depriving vulnerable community members who used to eat at ritual events of an important source of food.

Community leaders also reported that behaviour at the funerals themselves had changed, with people no longer talking to each other; and receiving take-aways instead of sitting and eating with the family. The role of community leaders at funerals had also changed, in part due to fear—"I go to funerals because I must be seen there, but leave early because I am scared of this thing [Covid-19]"; and in part due to difficulties in getting around: "I narrate the *umlibo* (genealogy) for the family, but only if the funeral is near." Community leaders also took some responsibility for announcing the rubric of the rules, such as the 50-person limit at funerals, although the general feeling was that it was not their responsibility to prevent people from attending: "That is a job for the police." When considering ways of improving the prevention of Covid-19, particularly in relation to funerals, a number of traditional, religious and community leaders noted that most of the communication had been via television and radio broadcasts. They recommended greater on-the-ground engagement from officials in rural areas, educating people about the rationale behind some of the rules, such as those for encasing bodies in plastic and preventing families from seeing the bodies, which were described as hard to understand. It was also recommended that the government should involve local people more in the decision-making around the rules that should be promoted and how they should be enforced. As one religious leader said: "The rules would have been more effective if local inputs had been sought. There should be more consultation to understand the different dynamics at lower levels."

Traditional and community leaders and ward councillors also indicated limited information sources for educating local people about the steps to prevent the spread of Covid-19; local traditional leaders were described as hustling for knowledge. One community leader indicated that no campaigns or training had been conducted to raise awareness locally. A councillor said the government had fallen short on teaching people, and recommended the production and dissemination of pamphlets. The leadership groups expressed divergent views on the extent and functionality of their communication with the government about the outbreak and its management. Some religious and traditional leaders were looking for greater involvement in government decision-making, although traditional leaders also reported relatively clear lines of communication with the municipality. Even ward councillors, who were clearly more connected to government systems like the office of the premier, described official responses as sluggish: "emails are sent but government is apathetic". For one religious leader, part of the challenge was how public communications had apparently become shaped by political concerns—"they are blaming each other". Considerable cynicism was also expressed about apparent double standards in the responses of the political class to the outbreak. For example, one community leader noted that while the funerals of poor people were strictly controlled, a recent local funeral of a leading official's relative had proceeded undisturbed.

In relation to practical efforts to stem the spread of Covid-19, including at funerals, local leaders were quite scathing about the shortfalls in government actions. One ward councillor baldly stated: "government interventions have failed", citing water shortage and the closure of a local clinic due to a lack of PPE. The theme was taken up by traditional leaders, who called for more protective equipment and materials—not just at funerals, where the municipality was obliged to provide 20 litres of sanitiser, but also to enable chiefs and kings to conduct their daily rounds and receive visitors safely. It was also noted that gravediggers should be provided with proper PPE, and a stakeholder workshop on PPE and sanitiser was proposed. There were also calls, including among community leaders, for the government to test many more members of rural communities, whose marginalisation from mainstream services rendered them particularly vulnerable to Covid-19.

More broadly, local leaders indicated that one way of responding to the present funeral regulations was to regard them as a "temporary arrangement". Some rituals could simply be postponed to a post-Covid-19 era, such as the hanging of jackets in church, and remedial action could be taken in future to rectify the cultural damage being done now. However, many leaders also indicated that there could be significant room for adapting the rules relating to the handling of bodies and funerals; in this way local people's cultural and psychological needs could be met while also preventing the spread of Covid-19. They found clear benefits for poorer people in trimming the time and expense of funerals, and even framed the new, simpler practices as a return to the old ways. In addition, certain customary practices were viewed as having taken on new meaning—such as the ritual washing of hands upon returning from the grave. Meanwhile, community members themselves were portrayed as having shown considerable flexibility—for example, using mechanical diggers in place of human ones. Leaders also felt they were prepared to negotiate around the issue of access to and contact with the bodies of their loved ones.

Several clear proposals seem to have emerged from this willingness, including a clear need to view and communicate with the body at the mortuary, and again once it had been brought home. It was also suggested that the current practice of the bodies being dressed by the morticians at the funeral parlour could be adapted to include family members. Meanwhile, strategies were adopted by mourning families to avoid ensuring adherence to attendance limits at funerals—such as holding funerals early before officials can arrive. They were concerned not with a lack of understanding of the need to contain and track the virus—for example, one religious leader reported that bereaved families had taken it on themselves to establish attendance registers and provide sanitisers and masks—but rather the socio-cultural difficulty of separating one's life from that of the community.

Gravediggers

The seven gravediggers who were interviewed for the study reported a number of challenges faced by local rural communities. According to one gravedigger, incomes had been slashed as the sale of surplus produce from the harvest became difficult under lockdown; another noted the impacts of the outbreak and the restrictions on communal socio-economic support networks: "Things are worse because you cannot go to your neighbour and ask for something because you are scared."

At the same time, the rules on physical distancing and mask-wearing were regarded as quite ineffective—for example, because of overcrowding in local taxis. A further significant problem reported was the lack of testing, which was seen as only available for those with money. Gravediggers are members of the rural communities they serve, and they reported that they had changed their practices at funerals as a result of the new regulations. The number of local volunteers for gravedigging had decreased because of health fears although the gravediggers leading the teams said they could not refuse to work—"we have to do our jobs".

To protect themselves, the gravediggers had taken a number of steps. They ensured that no more than two people, and in some cases only one, dug the grave at a time. They also divided their efforts among themselves—"now we split up, we do not all go to all the funerals". One gravedigger also reported that the digging was divided between families "to avoid crowds". The gravediggers expressed concern about the need to protect themselves from the spread of the virus, particularly in terms of handling tools. One reported: "We use one pick and one spade which now we must sanitise, but we do manage to maintain social distancing." However, another claimed that spades were shared, and no sanitiser was used since their hands were dirty. In a different case, it was reported that sanitiser was provided in the graveyard. Gravediggers identified a need for personal protective equipment, in particular gloves, which could be second-hand. The ritual washing of spades after the graves were dug had continued.

Many gravediggers felt the rules governing funerals should be observed; one emphasised that families should not hide the cause of death, "especially if the death was due to Covid-19". This was considered important, in part because people would then take the Coronavirus more seriously. Another gravedigger said he was now required to report funerals to the police. However, it was also acknowledged that despite community efforts to comply, the rules were being broken: "mourners cannot chase people away [from funerals]". Another respondent noted that when more than 50 people arrived for a funeral, the surplus numbers would go to a neighbour's place and attend from there. In addition, significant sympathy was expressed for the families of the deceased and their isolation from their communities as a result of the rules on numbers at funerals. Community and extended-family pressure to be part of the process was acknowledged:

> People try to comply but it is not easy. For example, when there comes a time for the body to arrive in the morning for burial, there is always that small prayer that usually happens before the ceremony starts, and people leave to go to the tent. The house where the prayer is done is usually small and there is no social distancing, and this is not by choice … One of the main reasons why people want to be part of the prayer is because many people want to see the deceased for the last time. So, it is difficult for the family of the deceased to control the line … it is difficult for people to accept that they cannot come and go as they please and that they cannot see the deceased for as long as they like.

Burial society members

The nine members of burial societies who were interviewed for the study described a number of social and economic challenges as a result of the outbreak and lockdown. They described "irresponsible" behaviour among youth and drinkers, who generally ignored physical distancing guidelines while they socialised. One respondent even noted that cultural dissonance had emerged around the issue of wearing masks:

> Some local people feel that you are using masks because you think they have the virus, when you are only protecting yourself and them in the process. They expect you to take off your mask, greet them, laugh with them, and at times hug them the same way we all did before the pandemic. When you don't want to socialise, they think that you are seeing yourself as better than them.

Respondents in this group also identified a number of vectors for the initial spread of the virus, such as Chinese people, including local traders; visitors from the cities; and funerals. The sense of social dissolution described was seen as having been amplified by the restrictions, which prevented tribal authorities and burial societies from meeting and led to churches being shuttered. Burial society members also reported that were no longer able to emotionally support bereaved families by visiting them and saying prayers to provide comfort. Now, only one or two senior members of the society would visit the bereaved to deliver groceries, or increasingly just money. In some cases, a car was hired to deliver food to the family, while the burial societies relied on cellphone banking to make payments to families and funeral parlours. In addition, burial society members were increasingly unlikely to attend the family funerals of other members. The changes of behaviour that had been adopted in adherence to lockdown measures were viewed as upsetting, as one burial society member explained: "We are hurt because it seems as if we do not care for one another because we are no longer giving full support to our members." The burial society members' views of the rules on funerals seemed largely shaped by prudence. The respondents noted that the new rules prevented families from spending too much money, which left more for their own use. In addition, it was noted that a distinction should be made between cultural practices, such as washing the gravediggers' tools, which would be followed regardless, and other actions prohibited under the rules—such as filling tents with visitors and producing programmes with many speakers—which were deemed unnecessary and "not culture". In this regard, families had also adopted a flexible approach to manage the numbers at funerals, even leaving to make space for a visiting community member since "it is not easy to chase out community members that are at funerals as they are there to support the family of the deceased".

A number of these respondents recommended adherence to the rules in the common interest. Although concern was expressed that the deceased would haunt the living with requests that they be dressed and wrapped properly, in cases where the appropriate customs had not been followed, it was acknowledged that "when we comply with the regulations, it is not to please the government but to protect ourselves". The burial society members noted that many households had sanitisers, but also advocated fumigation in cases of Covid-19 deaths. They also sought the official provision of masks and PPE for frontline staff and at gatherings, with one local woman already making and distributing masks for free at local meetings.

The police as enforcers of the law

In terms of the Coronavirus rules and regulations, the police force had a central role to play as enforcers. All deaths during this period needed to be reported to the police station and they were expected to monitor the behaviour at funerals. Death certificates could also be issued by a senior police official or a local magistrate. Seven police officers, including one detective, shared their views on the outbreak, the government's lockdown measures, and how these had changed their roles, including in relation to funerals. They indicated that the virus' spread had initially been blamed on Chinese people; migrants from Cape Town who had travelled to rural areas without knowing the outcome of Covid-19 tests that they had taken; and funerals. They affirmed the view that rural areas had been neglected by official responses to the outbreak: "food parcels on television went to people in towns but not here". They also expressed cynicism about the government's intentions of relaxing lockdown restrictions at the end of the first wave: "the government just opened taverns and churches to divert the focus of the people". Another claimed: "the government is now more concerned with making money than protecting the people."

Although the police reported some improvement in adherence to the rules as lockdown measures eased, there was widespread scepticism about the effectiveness of the restrictions and the police's own role in enforcing them. Respondents reported widespread flouting of the rules on physical distancing and mask-wearing, despite the police's efforts to publicise these via loudhailers in towns when local residents collected their social grants. In particular, rural residents were viewed as recalcitrant, with a number of officers reporting mounting hostility among this group. This was in part a result of police efforts to enforce the advice on physical-distancing and mask-wearing, as well as the regulations on funerals. Some police complained that they had been stigmatised for carrying out their duties, saying "that is why people always see us as their enemies", including at funerals: "people seem to think that police attend these funerals to make sure that everything is messed up". The police identified a number of specific issues around law and order that had arisen from the outbreak and lockdown. These included the men refusing to accept the regulations on the production and consumption of liquor, particularly older men brewing their own beer; cases of domestic violence that had either been caused by drinking at home or by women being blamed for not providing for their families; the frequent reported cases of Covid-19 regulations being contravened; a significant drop in arrests as residents avoided visiting police stations in town, where the virus was viewed as most prevalent; and widespread resistance to police enforcement of the rules, which was viewed as the result of a lack of effective public education about the impacts of the virus and how it is spread.

The police also expressed concern at the threat posed to their own well-being by the outbreak. One said that a local police commander had refused to extend help to sick people who needed emergency transport for fear that his officers could contract the virus. Another told a contrasting tale of his commander continuing to work after testing positive for Covid-19, prioritising the fight against crime over the health threat to his subordinates. Police told of being forced to work while sick; having to conduct searches and arrests without gloves and on mask-less suspects; travelling four to a car due to a lack of resources; and lacking the PPE required to do their jobs properly. For example, one officer said that he hadn't even been equipped with sanitiser to disinfect his handcuffs after they had been used to arrest a suspect. However, in another district, the police were reportedly equipped with gloves and sanitisers and their vans were frequently fumigated. In addition, it was noted that some awareness-training on the pandemic had been conducted. One particularly striking claim was that the number of police in quarantine had reduced the numbers on duty—this fact was reported to be widely known among local communities, which had encouraged them to blatantly flout the lock-down rules.

In relation to funerals, the police said their role was to check with funeral parlours that they had the necessary PPE and were following the rules. They were also charged with visiting the homes of the deceased to make sure they had sanitiser. They would attend the funeral to make sure that masks were being worn; physical distancing was being observed in the layout of the chairs; a register had been provided; and the numbers did not exceed 50. However, as one officer noted: "We do not know if people continue to comply with the rules after we have gone." In a similar vein, one of the officers said that compliance was only enforced on the day of the funeral and not before, for example, on the eve when the family may hold a night vigil: "there are more people that go to the house of the deceased before, than the actual day of the funeral". Another respondent noted the practice of starting funeral services early. In one case, the event took place from 4 am; by the time the police responded at 9 am to a complaint about the numbers at the event and its length, it was too late. The congregants were already leaving "and they were laughing".

This discourse of recalcitrant mourners strategising to break the rules at funerals was a common one among the police who were interviewed. One said families no longer reported deaths to avoid visits from police checking on their adherence to the protocols to prevent Covid-19. Another reported that the 50-person limit on funerals was widely broken—"I have not heard of a 51st person being turned away." It was also claimed that one close relative who had gone to the mortuary to view a body had dared the police to arrest her for risking her own life so that she could say goodbye to her loved one. One recurring claim was that wealthy, well-connected mourners enjoyed relative impunity at funerals given the difficulties faced by junior officers in enforcing the rules at these events. More broadly, the police perspectives on the impacts of the funeral rules on bereaved families were mixed. It was noted that quick funerals reduced the risk of contagion—particularly since "at least one of the family of the deceased may have it". In addition, one officer asserted: "if this is treated according to our culture many people will open these Covid-19 bodies, leading to more infections, meaning Covid-19 and culture cannot be mixed."

At the same time, there was scepticism about the value and utility of the restrictions on funerals. One officer referenced the common fear among bereaved families that if the body was not buried properly, it would have to be exhumed and re-buried "because the deceased will appear in their dreams or the ancestors will not be happy". This respondent advised that at least two members of the family should be allowed to see the body to make sure it was the right one. Another officer gave warning that "too many restrictions" on funerals would not slow the spread of the Coronavirus. "Funerals have to happen, and people have to attend them especially members of the family of the deceased. Also, they need support during funerals—and support in our communities is not only financial." The police also made recommendations about the funeral protocols and public safety and education. They emphasised the need for PPE for all front-line service providers, and also for the families of the deceased so they could attend and identify the body at the mortuary. It was also advised that family members should be allowed to talk to the body in line with their cultural beliefs. It was further recommended that greater efforts be made to educate people about Covid-19 and its spread—and not by the police, who were not trained to safeguard people's health and were anyway often seen as "enemies". Instead, they felt that health officials and funeral parlour staff should be properly trained to manage Covid-19 and inform and educate families about the virus and its spread. These workers and community leaders should be supported by adequate communications from the government.

In addition, respondents said the toll-free numbers and email contacts produced by the government to support its public education campaign should be disseminated more effectively. Some police suggested that a Coronavirus prevention unit could be established to monitor and enforce popular compliance with the Covid-19 regulations. Others said that the top-down communication strategy was not working and advised that greater efforts should be made to facilitate bottom-up communications and improve responsiveness to concerns. Although the evidence suggests that police generally took a hard line against customary practice, a number of case studies were recorded where the police displayed considerable discretion and sensitivity in their approach to their duties. They turned a blind eye to activities where prominent local families were involved and the regulations were not closely followed, or entertained requests to informally expand the number of mourners or lengthen the time of services. There was always, of course, the danger that they could be reported for bending the rules, especially if they applied the law differently in different cases in the same areas.

The funeral parlours and the law

In addition to the South African Police Services, Covid rules and regulations were enforced through the funeral parlours. Virtually all black South African families have some form of funeral cover to release funds to families so that they can pay for the rising cost of funerals and attend to the requirements of dignified burial. We discussed the escalating costs and the commodification of funeral services and packages since the end of apartheid in chapter four, where we referred to the massive death industry that arose in southern Africa during the AIDS pandemic, beginning in the 1990s at the time of democracy. As most families needed to access funeral insurance to cover the costs, the funeral parlours were an important resource for the enforcement of government policy. One part of the system of control was the police's active involvement in certifying death and monitoring funerals. The other key component was ensuring that the funeral parlours administered their services to the letter of the law—in other words, that they did not allow families to tamper with the bodies or impose a customary ethos over what was now meant to be a tight technical process of burying bodies swiftly and under strict sanitary conditions. Some of the most hysterical scenes observed in rural areas during the first phase of Covid occurred when funeral parlour staff arrived in hazmat suits with spray canisters to either sanitise houses ahead of funeral gatherings, or the grave site to ensure that bodies were hygienically buried. At the beginning funeral parlours were less prominent because the police were the primary enforcers in the rural areas, but when the death rate rose sharply from June, they were seen all over the region and were even more remote and inaccessible than the local political elites and police.

The seven funeral parlour employees we interviewed indicated that relationships between themselves and the families of the deceased had become strained due to fear and concerns over the handling of the bodies. In one case, it was reported that fear of Covid-19 had led families to abandon the bodies of the deceased into the hands of the undertakers, while local community members kept their distance from the funeral parlours' branded hearses. In other cases, however, family and community members insisted on opening coffins, viewing bodies and preparing them despite the rules against this, which the funeral parlour staff were supposed to enforce: "Even during this time of corona, the community still insists that they handle the body themselves and do what they need to do on the body." One respondent, however, said that people were now responding well to the new rules, although they did not like them, "because all people are treated the same. Corona or not corona, bodies are wrapped in plastic." The undertakers reported their efforts to ensure that family and community members followed the rules both at the parlour and during funerals, including at the graveside. One parlour placed the bodies of those who had died of Covid-19 in separate cold storage, while a number of respondents had only allowed two family members to view the body for identification purposes. Parlours reported giving staff the appropriate equipment and clothing to protect them while handling corpses and coffins. Staff said they also gave local pallbearers gloves to wear; brought sanitiser into people's yards for their use; and encouraged people to follow physical-distancing guidelines at funerals. They also noted that their role at funerals, which were now shorter, had been reduced. They acknowledged that their efforts to ensure compliance with the regulations were not always successful, in particular those relating to attendance registers, numbers at funerals and physical distancing. In this regard, one respondent noted that the autonomy of the family of the deceased should be respected more—"it is they who must decide what needs to be done with the body as a family".

Undertakers reported that the outbreak and lockdown regulations had been bad for business. People were buying cheaper caskets, which had previously been a major source of revenue. The shorter three-day time frames for burials had also posed logistical challenges, particularly in processing insurance claims to pay for the funerals. Some parlours were thus asking for advance payments from families, while others were fronting the money. In addition, the payment of regular instalments to funeral parlours had become a challenge for some families, who were afraid of going into town to make these cash deposits. It was advised that the parlours could accordingly make greater use of electronic banking services. A further financial concern related to the cost of the PPE, which was being provided by undertakers to family members who visited the parlours, as well as to other visitors such as officials and insurance company staff. Staff said the government should subsidise the cost of this PPE, which the undertakers felt unable to pass on to their cash-strapped clients. Undertakers noted a lack of communication between the government and the funeral parlour industry "unless there is something that requires our attention". In addition, staff complained that health department officials had issued a series of contradictory, shifting instructions on funerals.

One data-capturer for funeral insurance claims and application and another funeral insurer were also interviewed. The data-capturer indicated the importance of strictly following protocols to seal Covid-19 bodies "to avoid disadvantageous situations". The procedure was for the bodies which had tested positive for the virus to be wrapped at the hospital and subsequently tagged by funeral parlour staff, who did not see the body. "No one fiddles with the body, no one washes or changes them." Any clothes brought by the family were laid next to the bagged corpse in the coffin. The rules dictated that the body had to be taken still sealed to the graveyard on the day of the funeral and put in the ground. If the test results of a body that had already been wrapped came back negative, the plastic was removed and the body was washed before being passed to the undertaker. However, for Covid-19 cases, the last time that the family saw the deceased was when they were still alive at the hospital—once they died, no one was allowed to see or touch them. The insurance company representative considered the 50-people limit at funerals to be harsh for some families and also advised that the plastic wrapping should be transparent, or that mortuaries should offer coffins with a glass lid to enable viewing of the body. The representative also warned that the mobile cold storage used by the company to store Covid-19 bodies was full to capacity and that the lack of space could lead to the identities of the bodies being confused.

In August 2020, Carl van der Riet, Chief Operating Officer of Avbob, the largest funeral insurance company in South Africa, acknowledged that attendee restrictions on funeral services and the close monitoring of bodies had affected the South African people. He suggested that the funeral parlours and insurance companies regretted the trauma caused but had to apply the law otherwise they would lose their licences, acknowledging that:

> people process trauma in different ways and people rely on family networks to assist them and support them through times of bereavement like this. And that's, you know, the one potential area of impact

171

is that people no longer have that level of support and are no longer able to process trauma.[8]

Conclusion: Covid, community and class

Many community members whose views were canvassed indicated that they had felt abandoned to their fate at both the regional level—by the political and traditional leadership—and at the local, municipal and national levels by the government They reported absent leaders—for example, a traditional leadership that preferred to engage through local proxies rather than in person, or distant councillors—and a damaging bureaucratic disengagement, for example, as local home affairs offices were shuttered. In general, it was reported that many traditional leaders and political leaders with co-morbidities had abrogated their duties for fear of contracting the virus and losing their lives. Frontline staff, such as nurses and police officers, complained that they lacked the materials and support to provide proper services. Their fears for their own health led to many offering a lower level of service. At the same time, funeral parlour workers and other staff employed in the business of death tended to promote over-rigorous compliance rather than engaging with the concerns of bereaved families, for fear of transgressing complex, shifting rules, which, they claimed, had been poorly communicated. Anecdotal evidence also suggests that over-rigorous compliance may have stemmed from their own fears of contracting the virus. Meanwhile, community members with responsibilities to directly support the families of the dead continued to perform their duties while facing great risk. Gravediggers were stoic about the need to do their jobs. Priests expressed great awareness of the personal jeopardy in which they were placed when comforting the bereaved and conducting funerals, but continued through their sense of obligation to their congregations: as one said, "this is our service". In fact, five local priests were reported to have died during the research, including one who contributed valuable perspectives to this book.

This chapter has reported on the roles of community leaders and the various gatekeepers involved in the renegotiation of funerals during the first wave of Covid in the rural Eastern Cape. Strikingly, these narratives suggest that the paternalism of the state was largely endorsed at the local level by local politicians, policemen, clinical nurses, funeral parlour personnel and even some high-ranking traditional leaders. The arrogance of the regional bureaucratic rural petty bourgeoisie, as Roger Southall once labelled this class,[9] is nothing new in the former homelands. Under colonialism, a surrogate class was created with the capacity to operate at an arm's length of the rural poor; this was reenforced during apartheid. The post-apartheid settlement elevated many in bureaucratic jobs to the ranks of the new political regime; they have generally remained the key gatekeepers in rural areas. Rural elites are used to presiding over poor families with low levels of accountability. They also understand the need to remain loyal and obedient, and to properly understand the hierarchies of power that emanate from the centre to the periphery. This was first taught to them under ethnic national development. The existence of this rural class dimension, which has been entrenched with the growth of suburban nationalism and consumerism in the rural areas, has further deepened symbolic currencies of rural class formation. In this context, the opportunities for the emergence of Richards' "people's science" and regimes of care and prevention have been limited by local-level class differentiation and the political culture of the region, which has deep historical roots from the apartheid and colonial eras.

In West Africa, MSF was able to break down the hegemonic, top-down Western bio-medical approach by working with intermediaries, including secret burial societies, chiefs, and anthropologists. They developed an appreciation of the need for community engagement to improve care and prevention to contain and manage the Ebola virus. In the rural Eastern Cape and other homeland areas, the entrenched national bio-medical model, first strengthened during the AIDS pandemic, was articulated with political patronage and social and status differences to restrict the possibilities of "people's science" during the first phase of infection. This is, of course, not to suggest that more engaged and cooperative approaches will not emerge in future, but rather to note the ways in which the pandemic seems to have enhanced rather reduced community and class division. In the next chapter, we explore how families and communities increasingly took matters into their own hands after the first wave to address spiritual insecurity and cultural indignity.

6

EXHUMING BODIES

Introduction

In South Africa's rural areas, hopes of state support and protection during the first wave of Covid-19 had already been shattered by June 2020, when the first wave deaths peaked in the Eastern Cape. Fear and chaos engulfed the public health system as villages were traumatised by burying bodies in plastic bags. The new measures, which included tough restrictions on funerals, had initially been endorsed by traditional leaders who were eager not to break ranks with the ruling party and their state of disaster, imposed in March 2020 with guidance from the Ministerial Advisory Committee (MAC) on Covid-19. However, the reality of implementing the new measures and the state's war on funerals and customary practices left rural communities battered and confused because the protocols and practices which had been introduced to control funerals were culturally offensive and spiritually unsustainable. This was no way that a government sensitive to people's cultural rights and beliefs should be acting. Indeed, the measures associated with the plasticisation of bodies were introduced without a thorough investigation of the infectiousness of Covid-19 bodies, or any broad consultation with local communities and traditional leaders. The authoritarian "state of exception" mode of governance adopted by the regime sought to earn legitimacy from the global community by standing behind a hard-line, bio-medical, modernist approach, copying regulatory frameworks from the global North and pathologising customary practices. The blank rejection of customary practices as dangerous and problematic made it difficult for the state to work within rural cultural values and behaviours to find common ground and develop joint preventative strategies, as occurred during the Ebola epidemic in West Africa in the early 2010s.[1] The ruling elite's dismissal of customary practices as threats to public health also created a barrier between the state and traditional healers, who were deliberately left out of all discussion and strategies concerning the managing of Covid-19. The state seemed determined to dispel any perception that it was open to any approach other than Northern bio-medical science.

The state's tough approach left rural communities across the country in a state of shock, not only because of the devastation wrought by the Coronavirus in relation to their livelihoods and homes, but also as a result of their loss of faith and belief in the South African state and its services. In the 2016 local government elections, the Zuma presidency had managed to increase support for the ruling African National Congress (ANC) in rural areas.[2] However, by the 2019 national elections he had been replaced as party and national leader by Cyril Ramaphosa, a prominent urbanite businessman and former labour leader who came to power partly because of accusations of endemic graft within the state under Zuma's watch. Ramaphosa was from a minority ethnic group and did not appear to be an ethnic nationalist, nor did he seem to be as close to traditional leaders and customary concerns as Zuma had been.[3] His predecessor had in fact often warned rural communities that they should not take everything they received from the state, such as their pensions and welfare cheques, for granted because not every party and president would value them as much as he did. It was partly a threat, but also a powerful election ploy to retain the rural vote. Ramaphosa had a different profile, as an urban capitalist who spent relatively little time in the countryside and former homelands. He was generally perceived as a distant figure in the rural Eastern Cape; someone who represented the urban elites more than he did the rural poor. It was in this context that the rural poor interpreted some of the trauma of the first wave. They claimed that the

President had promised to look after all citizens equally but felt that the party now cared "too much for the urban people" and especially the middle classes in the city.[4] Many comments were also made after the televised funerals of ANC urban elites, who were apparently buried without plastic covering their bodies, proper social distancing or clear restrictions on the number of attendees. People were shocked to see that the coffin of Jackson Mthembu, the Minister in the Office of the Presidency, was not wrapped in plastic when he died in January 2021. They said that the very Office of the Presidency which was instructing them to forsake their customs did not follow its own rules.

Although the state claimed that everyone would be protected in the national "war" on Covid and that "no-one would be left behind", the rural poor felt abandoned, marginalised, and forgotten. They said that rural healthcare services could not cope with the pandemic and that the nurses there were not trained in Covid care. There were also frequent mentions of the absence of any public education on the virus, including in the home language of the region's Xhosa speakers. But most of all they complained about how their own customary practices and burial rites were undermined by a government that was "fighting with our traditions" rather than harnessing those traditions in the fight against Covid.[5] This chapter focuses on the period after the first wave, as the provincial government and local stakeholders came to play a greater role in the management of the pandemic in rural area, and communities themselves started to respond to the impact of lockdown on their cultural identities and spiritual well-being. As the provincial death rate was spiking during the first wave in July 2020, the Premier of the Eastern Cape, Oscar Mabuyane, introduced a set of new measures to contain the hysteria that Covid deaths and funerals were causing. He declared that provincial hospitals were required to declare deaths as a Covid death or not and record the cause of death on the official death certificate. This was a controversial intervention because, while it aimed to minimise the trauma of wrapping all bodies in plastic, families did not want the cause of death to be known. Covid, like HIV and AIDS, carried a negative stigma.[6] Some villagers interpreted the Premier's ruling as a deliberate attempt to expose families to shame and derision, by picking out the Covid deaths for special attention. They spoke of how Covid was associated with a stigma similar to AIDS in villages, although others said that the measures were sensible. The Premier also confirmed the regulations about wrapping Covid bodies and coffins in plastic and ruled that funeral services were limited to one hour to minimise interaction and infection. The Premier wanted to move away from an approach that seemed to blame custom for Covid to a more targeted approach, which focused on Covid deaths and minimised the fear and hysteria that gripped the villages.

The new provincial level regulations did not replace the national Disaster Management Act. They simply added an addition layer to the regulations which applied specifically in the Eastern Cape. The aim of the new provincial approach rules was to address the cultural, psychological, and spiritual shock of Covid deaths in rural areas by stopping funeral parlours from treating all bodies in the same way, while at the same time tightening the restrictions on Covid funerals.[7] The new rules were a response to the rising death rate but also to to the growing trauma of death in the rural areas, and criticism from within the provincial government and its stakeholders, which included the House of Traditional Leaders. However, by August 2020, local people's fear of the virus fell away naturally as the peaks of the first wave passed and the number of cases dropped. Tight lockdown was gradually removed, although the regulations governing funerals and customary practices remained in place. For the next three months people could move around freely as the province and the country tried to reopen-up for business. Urban migrants that had stayed at home in the rural areas after Easter could return to the cities, and those in the cities who had lost loved ones could come home to visit their families. Alcohol, which had been banned for months, was now also back on sale as rural life started to return to some sense of normality. However, ritual life and customary practice still did not return to the countryside. Ultimately, this pause proved to be nothing more than a lull before the storm. By late November, the second wave had started amidst outcry that a new South African variant, which originated in the Eastern Cape, was spreading globally. By the middle of December, the province buckled under the new wave as the death toll in the region allegedly reached as high as 500 per 100,000, especially in the two metros.[8] As cemeteries filled in the cities and families returning to their home villages were greeted by scenes of multiple deaths and daily funerals, fear once again gripped the province. At this time, local hospitals reported that the average Covid patient was dying within 48 hours of being admitted.[9] Most of the intensive care units in the province lacked adequate oxygen and were understaffed. The Eastern Cape had become the South African killing field for Covid.[10]

Meanwhile, the families of those who had died in the first wave were suffering in the knowledge that their loved ones had been interred in plastic bags and been buried without dignity, or trapped away from home where they were unable to complete their journey to the afterlife. The spiritual anxieties of these mourners were heightened by the new wave of death. This added to the existing problems in rural areas, including the difficulty of securing basic services like acquiring death certificates, Covid welfare grants and basic healthcare from the state. As people were now dying in large numbers and the state had obviously failed to protect rural citizens and strengthen local resilience, families increasingly took matters into their own hands and

Diagram 3: Excess deaths in the Eastern Cape

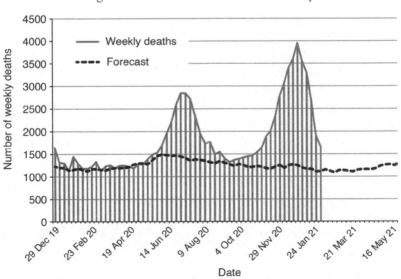

Based on data from the South African Medical Research Council.

began to defy government rules, especially in relation to customary practices. The focus of this chapter is on the response of rural families to the relaxation of lockdown rules from August 2020 and the measures they took to address the damage and indignity of Covid funerals. The chapter shows how, despite the Premier's intentions to add a provincial layer to the national regulations, local stakeholders— including chiefs, the police and councillors—were increasing open to hearing families' requests for special concessions. This meant that there was some capacity for manoeuvre at the local level after the first wave subsided. Following this discussion, the chapter focuses on the December 2020 home-comings from the cities, which occurred under the shadow of the second wave. Here we emphasise how the reunification of migrant families at home resulted in a surge of cultural resistance and defiance across the rural areas, as families started exhuming some of the bodies buried during the first wave and illegally reburied them in private ceremonies. We also discuss the return to customary practices like initiation ceremonies in December, after traditional leaders withdrew their support for an extended lockdown on custom.

The national state in retreat: Paternalism and panopticons

The appetite of the South African state to maintain martial law subsided when infection levels dropped in August 2020. Police withdrew from the villages and were less conspicuous at funerals and on street corners in rural towns. The general belief in the rural areas was that Covid had hit them like a tsunami but had now passed, and everyday life would gradually return to normal. Anxiety over the burial of kin in plastic bags remained a major topic of discussion in the villages, but as the death rate dropped the injustice seemed less ubiquitous; there were fewer funerals. As Covid restrictions had been followed in the region as a response to the fear of being arrested and charged, rather than through any significant local appreciation and understanding of the nature of transmission, the declining death rate and dramatically reduced number of cases opened the way for low levels of protocol adherence. As one man explained:

> People were watching for the government and the police. They were doing this thing out of fear not out of free will. They would wear

masks and socially distance when they thought they were being watched by people who could report them or directed by the police. I would take the taxi into town to do shopping. There was not much mask observance in the village but by the time I arrived in the queues at [the] store in town, there were police around, and most people were wearing masks. The rules about limiting the number of passengers in taxis were generally not applied nor were they enforced. It seems that the local police like to bully individuals but do not make trouble with powerful people like taxi bosses. I was also really shocked at the venom of the police blitz on funerals right at the beginning. There were at least two officers at every funeral and a van somewhere in the background. If things were not right, they would just tip pots of food and beer, and put people in the van. It was crazy because these guys were nowhere to be seen if someone was robbed or assaulted in the villages. They must have been threatened by their bosses about the funerals because I have never seen such attention to detail in the work of the police in rural areas.[11]

The passing of the first wave resulted in a weakening of central command. The state eased the lockdown in rural areas and allowed interprovincial travel, the sale of alcohol and access to public parks and places, such as beaches, which had formerly been out of bounds. However, none of the rules for funerals were changed, nor the ban on customary gatherings. Meanwhile, the Minister of Health, Zweli Mkhize, no longer performed the political rituals of dominance and control over the province, as he had at the height of the hard lockdown when he held national press conferences and castigated and disciplined local officials. Now the national government sought to work with provincial structures to ensure that the transitions from one level of lockdown to the next were understood and implemented in a uniform way, and that provincial departments and municipalities were staying alert. The decentralisation of control introduced a period of incrementalism, as local and provincial officials tried to tweak various rules and regulations to address local circumstances more effectively.

As the lockdown eased, President Ramaphosa also changed his tone and spoke less of his support for the police and the army in disciplining citizens, and more of the need for citizens to take greater responsibility themselves. He warned that, if they did not comply, he would not hesitate to re-introduce harsh and repressive measures. In the urban areas, he stressed the dangers of the sale of alcohol and constantly connected tavern life to township life. He emphasised that this had become a toxic conduit not only for the escalation of interpersonal and gender-based violence, but represented a space where people did not follow rules and did as they pleased.[12] To disconnect the township from its internal mimesis, the state constantly toyed with an alcohol ban and different possibilities and permeations thereof. In the period between August and December various options were explored and implemented, including a ban on alcohol sales and access to public spaces over Christmas, when the second wave was at its peak. In the rural areas, funerals and customary practices continued to attract constant attention in the media and in the speeches of the President and the Premier, who was increasingly making his own statements in relation to managing the provincial reality. The message was irrefutable and clear: funerals were deadly events and the bodies that arrived at them were toxic and highly contagious. The warning from the President was that, while the state no longer had the inclination to micro-manage every funeral, people would die in large numbers if they did not take charge of safety at these rituals and police themselves and their neighbours.[13]

The use of funerals as a kind of panopticon for rural self-discipline proved counter-productive in the absence of wider public health engagements among local leaders, health officials and rural people. It simply created more fear, which drove down attendance numbers. At the outset of the pandemic, it was difficult to restrict funerals to 50 people because under normal circumstances they would be large public gatherings and rituals that went on for two days, starting with the funeral services and then moving onto feasting and socialising. By the end of the first wave, and in the face of constant warnings about the danger of funerals and Covid bodies, attendance started to drop to well below the 50-person threshold. When people were asked why they did not like to attend burials anymore, they talked of their fear of catching Covid at these events, but also their concerns about eyes of the state and tell-tale neighbours and village do-gooders being upon them. One woman said: "One never knows who is watching at these events, you feel fearful that you will be reported and then be put in jail."[14] Another believed that the decreasing numbers were due to the constant threats from the President, which seemed to suggest that even though other activities could return to normal, funerals would remain under scrutiny. This created a panopticon effect, under which avoidance was driven both by the genuine fear people felt towards infectious bodies but also the hidden eyes of snitches and police informers in their midst. This was all made possible by the culture of fear instilled during the first wave of the pandemic. In addition to these considerations, there were simply too many funerals to attend during the second wave. Reports from the villages suggest that at least two or three burials were taking place every week, rather than one every other week. In some villages there were reports of funerals taking place every day during December and January, and even cases where 10 to 12 funerals were recorded in a single week. In this context, attendance dropped to only a handful of close kin, raising questions about the cultural legitimacy of the funerals as inclusive community events. This added to the pervasive sense of spiritual insecurity in the villages.

However, as numbers dropped at funerals, more resources were being diverted to what people call the "after tears parties", which often happen a week or two after the funeral. At these social events, mourners and friends gathered in a joyful celebration of the life of the deceased with food and alcohol, away from the sombre atmosphere of the funeral itself. The popularity of these events was partly attributed to the shortening of funerals to two hours; food prepared for the guests at the funeral was also not consumed on site but instead taken home in hampers. At best, the sharing of food after the funeral was curtailed to an hour or so. However, this was not a customary expectation and so the "after tears" parties gained great significance during the pandemic, especially after hard lockdown when it was easier to socialise in relaxed groups, away from the watchful gaze of the police. The "after tears" parties were also much more popular with the youth because alcohol was served there. According to Phila Dynatyi, rural-based youth and family embraced the "after tears" events because they did not want be near the body and were frightened to see the plastic wrappings and the undertakers in their hazmat suits.[15] He said that people found such scenes alienating and strange and just wanted a relaxed atmosphere to discuss and remember the deceased, as they would have at home before the regulations were introduced. Phila said that the popularity of these events was not just about people wanting to escape scrutiny but had a lot to do with their celebratory spirit in depressing times.[16]

Although traditional leaders took a back-seat at funerals during the first wave, often preferring to send more junior members of their clan or even local headmen in their place for fear of the own lives, they were nevertheless aware of what was happening in their villages. At a meeting of the House of Traditional Leaders in September 2020, several members, especially from the Bizana and Mthatha areas, noted that they had received numerous complaints from their followers about the way in which funerals were being conducted under Covid and the spiritual insecurity brought on by plasticisation of bodies, the shortened rituals and poor attendance. They reported that people were having worrying dreams which they viewed as connected to the traumatic burial conditions being imposed under Covid. One chieftainess from Bizana said:

> Villagers come to my place every week now with complaints about family members having bad dreams. They ask why the traditional healers are not around to help troubled families and why customary events, which might help them deal with the trauma, are not permitted. They are angry with us as traditional leaders for allowing the ANC to impose the current situation where people are buried in plastic. They say we have been taking a back-seat when communities are suffering.[17]

While the Eastern Cape House of Traditional Leaders did not want to be seen to defy the President or the Minister of Health, or the wisdom of Professor Salim Abdool Karim and his esteemed group of bio-medical scientists on the MAC, in this meeting they expressed the clear desire to see a return to normal customary practices as soon as possible.[18] They said that their communities needed them, and they wanted to intervene to support them. As a result, a gap started to emerge between the decisions at the central national level and the views of traditional leaders and their organisations, who complained about the regulations around burials and the lack of clarity on the future of customary practices, especially male initiations.

By September, the Congress of Traditional Leaders of South Africa (CONTRALESA) and the Eastern Cape House of Traditional Leaders had started to campaign to open the December season for male initiations. They claimed that it was not viable for the state to deny men the possibility of achieving manhood twice in the same year. As time passed and the December season grew nearer the voices of the chiefs, with the support of the provincial government, became ever louder, arguing for male initiation rituals to take place under controlled conditions. Professor Salim Karim and his team decided that an exemption was difficult to justify, given the social intimacy and high level of interpersonal contact involved, which was more than a large church gathering or service which remained banned. In the end, customary practices did resume in the rural Transkei in December, despite recommendations to the contrary from the MAC and the Office of the Presidency. Traditional leaders also said that families should be allowed to identify the bodies of their loved ones at mortuaries.

From secret burials to exhuming bodies

In view of the restrictions of customary funerals from March 2020, some traditional healers and leaders recommended that their people employ the strategy of temporary "secret burials" historically used by Xhosa people during wartime. In periods of crisis when a dignified burial was not possible, it was permitted for families to bury their loved ones temporarily, often just in a blanket, without notifying the community. In May 2020, the AmaMpondomise King in the former Transkei, Zwelozuko Matiwane, issued a ban on already-restricted traditional funerals and encouraged people to re-introduce the ancient practice of *ukughusheka*, or secret burial. His spokesperson, Chief Nkosi Bakhanyisele *Ranuga*, said that measure was taken to protect people spiritually and financially. Secret burials were cheap to perform and ritually sound because the family would make a ritual offering to the ancestors after the private burial to inform them that a proper funeral would occur later. He explained that: "when following this custom [of *ukuqhusheka*] this means people are called on to bury either on the same or the next day and with only those who were present at the time of passing".[19] Chief Ranuga said that a sacrifice to the ancestors after the immediate family had buried their loved one in a temporary grave would protect the family from "the dark cloud

185

of death".[20] The chief also explained that using the secret burial option spared families the cost of a traditional funeral at a time when there was no guarantee that such a ceremony would provide peace and spiritual security.

During the fieldwork underpinning this book, we found that a number of secret burials had taken place in the villages around the town of Engcobo in the Chris Hani district of the Eastern Cape, where large number of AmaMpondomise clans and families reside. In one case, an old man from a senior house in Sinqumeni rural village in Engcobo died in March. His death was not Covid-related but the family were not prepared to bury him under Covid restrictions because of his seniority. They felt that if a full burial was held, they would need to invite more than 50 people, slaughter several beasts for the ancestors and hold an event for longer than two hours to honour his life properly. In March the immediate family decided to instead do a secret burial, *uqhusheko lomzimba*, in the hope that a decent funeral, appropriate to his status would be held in the near future when the pandemic had subsided. The family members had believed that lockdown would last no longer than a month, and that after that, everything would be normal again for them "to bury their father in a decent way with traditions". When it became clear that the lockdown was not about to end soon, the family became anxious that their father might be angry and alone in his coffin in a shallow grave and decided to hold a Christian service for him. However, not everyone wanted to attend that event; some people preferred something more traditional since the clan was of royal descent. The whole event was unsatisfactory and a few weeks later, the deceased appeared in his daughters' dreams complaining of feeling cold and wet and that his head was not resting well in the coffin. In the dream, the man asked his daughter for her jersey to keep him warm. According to the family, the problem arose from the fact that the mortuary had not allowed them to dress the body before burial and that, in the rush to complete the secret burial, they had not attended to all the traditional details. In December 2020, the man was exhumed and reburied, following tradition and the orders his daughters had received in their dreams. The plastic wrapping on the coffin was removed and the jersey put in the coffin, while the plastic covering around the body was also removed because it made the dead man sweat and become wet.

The problem with secret burials, as the above case suggests, is that they were generally imagined as temporary affairs. In fact, sometimes the body was not even placed in a coffin but was just wrapped in a blanket because it was assumed that it would be exhumed and reburied in a matter of weeks. When this was not possible, families became stressed and often took matters into their own hands. Secret burials thus often created more problems than they solved. And the spiritual insecurity created by the Covid regulations were not only confined to the burial of senior men in the family, who required large and lavish funerals. More generally, the interruptions in customary practices created great cultural anxiety. For example, many mourners were concerned that their loved one's body did not spend the night in the home, where close kin could commune with it, and was instead simply dumped in the grave on the day of funeral. The legitimacy of funerals was limited by the bans on sacrificial offerings and communal eating and drinking; the time limits on funerals; the rules about social distancing; and the fact that the family could not dress the body before burial. But it was the plastic wrapping of bodies that created the most anxiety. Somadoda Fikeni, who is an expert on Xhosa and Mpondomise cultural practice, noted that traditional communities in the region were willing and able to adjust their customary practice in times of change, but the wrapping of bodies in plastic posed certain spiritual challenges that they found difficult to resolve.

By encouraged secret burial as a means of avoiding the indignity of Covid burial, the Mpondomise paramount opened the space in the north-western part of the former Transkei for families to start defying government rules and claiming back control of their own funerals. From August, when the lockdown measures were softened and travel was possible, there was a growing sense in the rural areas that action was needed to rectify some of the spiritual and reputational damage that had been caused by Covid funerals. The greatest sense of grievance was felt in homesteads where elderly men or women had died, usually of old age rather than Covid, and were exposed to the regulations that restricted attendance, cut back on the time allowed for the service, and denied villages access to the homestead or food during the proceedings. We recorded two burials in the Mbashe district around the town of Willowvale, where the seniority of the deceased clashed with the letter of the law. Neither of the individuals died of Covid, although both were over 75 years old. The main issue in both cases was the inflexibility of the rules, especially when esteemed elders were buried in the villages.

In the first case, an 82-year-old woman from a prominent clan passed away in May 2020. She was deeply respected and revered in the community and the expectation was that a full day ceremony would be held in her honour, with attendance from the entire village. However, the police insisted that the funeral should take no longer than two hours and that no more than 50 people could attend. They also ruled that food could not be served at the homestead and that the family would have to provide take-away lunches for the guests. The family complained bitterly, stressing the age and seniority of the woman involved, but no concessions were made by the authorities. On the day of the funeral, more than a hundred people gathered. Fifty stood outside the homestead to listen to the proceedings from a distance. There was grumbling about the register and the fact that only those on the list—the immediate family—were allowed to enter the premises. There was even more surprise when it was announced that only two members would speak at the funeral during the service. One man said that: "this was totally disrespectful and wrong; this woman has served her community with dedication. A life of that quality cannot be summarised in a few words".[21] The man claimed that: "I have seen criminals and people who died from gunshot wounds get more time than this".[22] The family made the same point and blamed the police for refusing to acknowledge that the hierarchies of life must be acknowledged in the rituals of death. As one family member put it: "these police are from this area, they should know better than to disrespect an elder in a family like ours".[23] The other case involved a slightly younger man from the same clan. He was a renowned community leader and elder, who died in August. But on this occasion the police allowed 75 mourners rather than the 50 permitted. They also allowed more time for speeches and for the food to be served on site to those in the yard.[24]

Both cases highlight the complex dynamics of status and hierarchy in rural areas and the offence people and families took to the insensitivity of the government rules to these aspects of rural life. The wrapping of bodies in plastic was intolerable to all the families, but so was the failure of the state to acknowledge the need for funerals to express social difference and hierarchy. But not everyone was prepared to accept the Covid regulations as these families in Willowvale did. In Engcobo we collected a case of a 78-year-old man who died in July shortly after the Premier had made his ruling that all death certificates should state whether the death was a caused by Covid or not. The man involved was a local schoolteacher and widely respected and known. He was a sickly man with chest problems, which stretched back more than a decade. However, when he fell ill and died in the hospital, his death was designated a Covid death. It appeared as such on the certificate. His family insisted that the hospital had made a mistake as he had no signs of Covid when he was admitted to hospital. They refused to change the form which made his wife and family extremely upset as they proceeded with the Covid burial and coffin wrapped in plastic. One of the family members said that the death certificate shamed the family and stigmatised her father, who had died from a pre-existing chest condition. It was a normal "natural death", she insisted, not something "caused unnatural cause, like AIDS or Covid".[25] Another family member said that the diagnosis seriously dishonoured the family by leaving the impression that he was careless and irresponsible in life. It left a smear on the family name, which apparently caused the mother to fall ill. The family connected the illness of their mother to the "smearing of the family name" and the manner of their father's funeral. The daughter also dreamt that her father felt trapped and claustrophobic in his sealed coffin. In August, less than a month after the funeral, the family decided to exhume the body, remove the plastic bags and bury the father in a private family ceremony.

At the reburial, family members declared their delight at having released the spirit of the beloved father and created the conditions for the mother to recover from her illness. This never happened, and she died a year later in July 2021.[26]

Public health beyond breaking point

Rural communities were critical of the role traditional leaders played during the first wave of the pandemic and how they had aligned themselves with the ruling urban elite's "state of exception" approach, offering their whole-hearted support for the lockdown measures and ban on customary practices. It was widely alleged that they had failed to champion the needs and concerns of the rural poor. Some chiefs and headmen in more remote areas and on the fringes of the ruling party alliance had also been angry about the lockdown rules and had tried to defy the ban on customary practices by keeping initiation lodges open or turning a blind eye. However, dissatisfaction with the traditional leaders increased as the Covid crisis deepened and rural communities failed to see any material benefits coming from the state. They also wondered why traditional leaders had taken a back-seat in community affairs and kept out of sight, even at important funerals where their presence was required. Rural residents felt deserted by their traditional leaders on the issue of the burial of plasticised bodies. They insisted that their leaders knew that this practice was unacceptable to the people but were saying nothing to challenge the rules, or even to explain why the measures were being taken in the first place. There was an eerie silence in rural areas for several months where nothing was being communicated. At a meeting in September 2020, several traditional leaders explained that they were alert to the spiritual crisis in their communities around the burial of bagged bodies but were unsure how they should handle it. They also felt that customary practices should be permitted because youths needed to be initiated and many families wanted to resume such rituals.

As the male initiation season approached at the end of 2020, the Eastern Cape House of Traditional Leaders and CONTRALESA increasingly petitioned the state to allow initiation rituals to take place and to lift the ban on customary practices. In October it seemed as if their wish would be granted, but when the first evidence of the second wave appeared in the Eastern Cape a month later there was heated debate about whether and how the annual initiations rituals might be conducted.[27] Male initiation rituals are conducted in two main phases: one when the boys go to the bush to be trained and circumcised by the *ncibi* (traditional surgeon) and another when they return to their home village for celebrations and gifts associated with their reintegration into the community. In the Eastern Cape, it was decided that the celebratory home-coming rituals should be suspended until after the Covid-19 pandemic had subsided. However, the boys were allowed to be trained and circumcised in the bush. Traditional leaders had to ensure that the first phase of the male initiation process took place with due consideration to social distancing and sanitisation.[28] Meanwhile, the national government, the provincial government and the House of Traditional Leaders did not make any rulings on other matters of ritual, which meant that other customary practices could now resume as normal with appropriate social distancing and sanitising in place. The ruling, together with the lifting of all restrictions on interprovincial travel, opened the door for families to start planning their home visits over Christmas and to schedule ritual activities involving family and kin. In addition to the issue of male initiation, potential rural reburials were a key concern for rural families over the Christmas period. The process of exhuming bodies and reburial was governed by legislation, as families were supposed to submit applications for approval before embarking on such activities. This was not how the families themselves generally approached the matter, and many made plans to rebury the bodies of their loved ones informally at night and in secret with only a small group of family members present.

Against the background of these policy shifts, the failure of the state to patch up the public health system, retain doctors and nurses and improve service delivery protocols in the months before the second wave produced even more disastrous outcomes in hospitals and clinics than the first wave had. The death rate in the Eastern Cape was higher than elsewhere in the world, exceeding 250 per 100,000. It was compounded by the ramshackle state of the provincial health service, which was suffering severe shortages of skilled staff in almost every area, as well as a general lack of medicines and equipment. The conditions in the sector were laid bare by a series of articles in the *Daily Maverick* entitled "A Province at Breaking Point". Senior health journalist Estelle Ellis anchored a team of investigators who traversed the province assessing issues of capacity, budget allocations, medical malpractice, rural clinic functionality, patient complaints and litigation against the Department of Health.[29] The series started with a description of the dire financial crisis at the provincial department of health, reporting how medical waste was building up at facilities because the department was unable to pay service providers. According to the lawyers, the department's unpaid bills amounted to R3.8 billion and a total of R37 billion in medico-legal claims had been made against it, which the department had no budgetary allocation for. Over 10% of the total 2021/2022 budget of R86 billion had already been spent on these claims before the year started; together with the R57 billion spent on salaries, this left the department with a miserly R10 billion for all other expenses, including medicines, maintenance, building costs, equipment maintenance, ambulances and other basic services.[30]

Turnover in the department's leadership had resulted in the appointment of three different provincial ministers during the Covid-19 pandemic, and high staff turnover only compounded matters. The main hospital for Covid patients in the province, Livingstone Hospital in Nelson Mandela Bay, had been headed by five different managers since 2018 and was understaffed in almost every department. The medical waste that had piled up here led to it being described as the "hospital from hell" by the BBC during the first wave. The *Daily Maverick* reported that, during the second wave, more than 40% of Covid-19 patients admitted to hospitals in the province wave died within 48 hours of arrival. This figure was even higher in the rural hospitals.[31] Most hospitals were death traps for patients, nurses and doctors, and were drenched in fear. The number of nurses who died on the job was also high because of the lack of protection offered in the hospitals;[32] and the level of mental illness among staff in these hospitals was high. Nurses who were interviewed for our study likened coming to work to playing Russian roulette, with bullets in more than half of the chambers. Phumla Mnyanda, who runs a 260-bed hospital in the Eastern Cape's capital, Bhisho, said that social media posts had spread misinformation on ways to avoid hospitals where people were dying. This stopped an even greater number of people from coming in when they first felt symptoms. But, as patients neared death, families would rush them to the hospital only to find that little could be done to save their relatives. "They were coming too late, and by then, their oxygen levels are very low, and you saw it dropping and dropping, and there is nothing we could do," she said in a telephone interview. "People are so scared because there are so many who have died."[33]

EXHUMING BODIES

Home-comings at Christmas time 2020

Like Easter, December is an important time for urban migrants to return home and reconnect with their families and home spaces. In the colonial and apartheid era, migrants flooded home at this time of the year because their nine-month labour contracts ended; because they needed to come home during the summer rainfall period to help plough and prepare the land for another season of crop production; or simply because they were tired and wanted to rest at home over the Christmas period. As previously noted, Ngwane argued against those who stressed the social cohesion of the homestead, suggesting that it was only really at Christmas time that rural households and families were united around a common purpose as domestic groups.[34] Easter may also be considered a moment when this affective economy of rural home-coming produces heightened emotions in support of togetherness. The traditions of home burial and territoriality, of fighting and suffering for home and for the integrity of the family and clan are deep-rooted and linked to specific places. It has also become increasingly common for families to socialise more generally with home people, as well as friends that they have made in the cities and at work, in towns along the coast in the Eastern Cape. The city of East London and the coastal town of Port St John's have become two destinations visited by many middle-class migrants. Home-coming, however, is certainly not just an exercise of social connections; it has always been a time of spiritual renewal, when men and women connect with their cultural roots and traditions in their places of origin and the landscape where their ancestors roamed.

One of the fieldworkers who contributed to this research, Zipho Xego in Bizana, found that families did not have the big family lunches and gatherings that would normally be seen around this season. Usually people from different families in different households would eat together or share food, even eating Christmas lunch together, but this year they spent Christmas in their houses. Xego explained:

> It is a "norm" in the village that on Christmas day, young children wake up, take a bath early in the morning and put on their new Christmas clothes. After breakfast, the children will walk in groups and will be going from house to house asking for "Christmas" in the

form of delicacies such as biscuits, sweets, and desserts. Adults also have activities that they indulge in. There is usually a dance setup that is known as *umdaniso*, which means "dance" in English. Here, people gather in a tavern set up with music, alcohol, and of course dancing being the main elements of the gathering. This often starts from 23 December and more or less continues everyday through to 2 January. It is always held in a neutral place, away from those places that sell alcohol in the area. and people bring their drinks. I remember, as a young girl, I once attended *umdaniso* even though I was underage and kids were not allowed. They allowed me as I entertained them with my dancing skills at the time. Kids usually hang outside the place as they cannot enter the place and it is the responsibility of those in attendance. This year things were slightly different in this sense. On Christmas day and building up to it, it was quieter than normal, people stayed in their yards, kids were not in the streets visiting people and their peers.[35]

Xego reported that people were too traumatised by the shock of the second wave to follow their normal social rituals and events this year. She noted that the general feeling of togetherness was not there in the villages because of the death and depression that Covid had brought. People were mortified that the government had prevented them from making their annual New Year's Day pilgrimage to the sea to wash off the previous year's misfortune and start afresh. She was particularly sad about this given the year many of her neighbours and friend had experienced:

> It is almost as if it is a norm that on 31 December people go to the beach to welcome in the new year. After all the festivities of the build-up to Christmas Day and after, the village is often quiet from 31 December as most people especially the youth go to the beach for the new year. They book taxis in advance and it is not strange to find that there will be two or three taxis operating from each area. I can recall when I was younger, this is what we were looking forward to as young people as a way of touching base with one another. Some of the people in the party would only go home once in a while. These were childhood friends and family members that one might only see over the festive season and all these get-togethers that people have. The coordination of beach trips takes place way before the festive season is in motion. The lobbying of who will be travelling with whom before the festive season is in full swing. The taxis are booked well in advance as people worry about not finding transport, as most

taxis get booked. Most of the time, these people do not even book accommodation, only the affluent will book accommodation and those will even travel with their transport. The rest of the group will sleep in the taxis and return the following night. This exercise serves the purpose of promoting belonging and togetherness among the people of the community, which is an important principle in the village. The beach trip also signifies the start of a new life. There is a common belief that is held by many, and that is, swimming in the ocean on New Year's Eve is a way of releasing and getting rid of the previous year's misfortune and cleansing oneself of bad omens to welcome the new year in a cleansed body that is ready to receive the new year's blessings.[36]

The experience of being at home in December is also about participating in family discussions about ritual and spiritual matters. Home-coming means planning for rituals for the future. In a survey conducted on rural homemaking in 2010 in the Transkei, involving 1,000 rural households in different areas, 33% of household heads said they would never consider moving away from their ancestral homes because "our ancestors are buried here".[37] A further 47% said they would not sell these homes because their families would not allow it, claiming that family land is not for sale. The same survey found that 553 households, or 53% of the sample, had performed a ritual at their homes over the previous three years, with the frequency of rituals varying from one to eight rituals. Overall, almost 1,000 rituals had been performed by the 553 households in the previous three years. In December, male initiation (*umgidi*) and the introduction of new-born children to the ancestors (*imbeleko*) were the most common rituals that were held. A related survey found that 42% of the cattle slaughtered in the former Transkei were killed for ritual purposes, rather than for family food consumption or the sale of the meat.[38] However, in 2020, the home-coming season was dominated by death rather than the pleasant, happy sounds of *umgidi* and *imbeleko* rituals in the villages or families feasting and dancing from Christmas to New Year. The cultural atmosphere was shaped by an almost daily procession of death and funerals, as families gathered by the light of day to bury new corpses, while others moved around under the cover of dark to exhume plastic-wrapped bodies and rebury them.

By the time the second wave broke in the Eastern Cape, there were several reports of families burying the wrong body and dreaming of the torture of their loved ones. In response, traditional leaders increasingly spoke out. In November, the CONTRALESA provincial chairperson, Chief Mwelo Nonkonyana, urged the government to forge a strategy to accommodate families wishing to view the bodies:

> They will talk to nobody else [besides themselves about this crisis]. They are not going to talk to any government official or to any leaders somewhere. They will talk directly to the families concerned, as to why you are not burying me. These things are real, and we do have real cases. A person from KwaZulu-Natal was nearly buried in the Eastern Cape, and a body from the Eastern Cape was buried in KwaZulu-Natal and had to be exhumed.[39]

Traditionalist Nokuzola Mndende weighed in on the debate, arguing that a body separated from the soul cannot be suffocated by layers of plastic:

> I don't think there is suffocation because the soul leaves the body. It goes to the spiritual world. That is our belief and wrapping the body with plastic for health purposes to avoid the spread of the disease is excellent. What I advise is that at least just to identify the body, the side of the plastic that is covering the face should be transparent.[40]

Meanwhile, funeral parlour owners in the Eastern Cape, such as Odwa Duru, expressed their concern:

> Quite honestly there is no way. We have to use three-layer plastic. Traditionally, I fully understand the outcry of the people, especially in the Eastern Cape. We do understand. I am Xhosa, I do rituals. I am also appeasing the ancestors. It's not nice, you know, to bury your loved ones, especially the father, mother, you take the body from the mortuary straight to the graveyard without taking the body or coffin to the *kraal* where we talk to the ancestors.[41]

In Goso village in Engcobo, a case was reported of a 60-year-old woman who contracted Covid-19 in August 2020 and was already unconscious when she was admitted to the hospital by her fearful family. She died in the intensive care unit. As her illness and death were very sudden, proper arrangements were not made for her burial, and the family was unsure whether to undertake a secret burial or conduct a full traditional ceremony. In the process, many stages in the normal ritual were missed or cut short, such as talking to the deceased before burial and the ritual dressing of the body (*unxibisa*). According to close kin, the ritual was a confused, inconsistent shambles. They were unsurprised that the woman then appeared in her children's dreams telling them that her spirit was wandering and did not know where it was going. In one of her daughters' dreams, she said that she had "not packed her wardrobe before leaving". The family felt she was implying that she had not found closure and that things had been left unfinished. In short, the burial rites had not performed the cultural work they were intended to enact, and for her spirit to rest, the funeral and burial would need to be redone. As in the previous case, the woman was eventually reburied in December 2020, when the family returned home for Christmas.

In a third case from the Engcobo area, the Faleni family in Nkwenkwana village exhumed the body of their father in January 2021. Thembisile Faleni was a taxi driver and the male head of the household, who had died of Covid in July 2020 and had been buried wrapped in plastic. Within weeks of his burial in the village, his widow, Nolusapho, said that her deceased husband started appearing in her dreams and the dreams of other relatives, complaining about suffocation caused by the plastic. The deceased also said that he was "tied up like a criminal". The dreams went on for months before Nolusapho called a family meeting to discuss them. The family decided that they would exhume and rebury him over Christmas when the family came home from the cities, so that he could rest in peace. They did this without informing the police or seeking permission from the government for the exhumation. His widow said "we decided to dig up his grave at night", with the help of 10 men, who "were shocked to discover he had been tied up and they removed the ropes". It is not clear whether she meant this literally or figuratively by referring to the plastic wrappings as "ropes". Interestingly, the case was reported through the media, indicating that the family did not care about being known to have broken the law. All they wanted was to end the hardship and torture that Thembisile had experienced because of the Covid rules on the plasticisation of bodies. Local traditional expert Loyiso Nqevu said they were concerned about the Covid-19 method of burial because "it neglects family values and customs". Nqevu said he knew of at least four families who had exhumed their loved ones, removed the plastic coverings and reburied them. He explained that: "according to our tradition, there is still life, even after death".[42]

Return to customary practice

In rural areas of the Eastern Cape between December and January 2020–21, the growing resistance towards the state regulations controlling funerals was accompanied by a return to customary practices in these areas. Many families performed rituals of healing and cleansing to address the insecurity of the Covid crisis. The family practices were also augmented by a general, though tentative, return of significant community rituals such as male and female initiation. Male initiation ceremonies had been officially suspended in April and there was general agreement that a second suspension in December would create serious problems with the uninitiated potentially roaming around rural areas.

Since the December and New Year holiday is generally the longest of the year, it is usually the time when most boys go to the mountain and when customary celebrations are performed in the communities. In 2020, the number of expected celebrations was further increased by pent-up demand for the performance of rituals which had not been possible during the first wave. By the time the second wave peaked over the Christmas holiday, anticipation had mounted among rural communities that long-delayed rituals could be observed, although the expectation was mixed with fear of the virus itself. Against this background of cultural anticipation, revised government regulations allowed initiation schools to open. However they had to observe Covid-19 regulations which included a ban on home-coming celebrations for initiates at the homestead. Young male initiates were allowed to stay at initiation schools (*amabhome*) for a sufficient period, as stipulated by custom; and traditional circumcision, or *ukwaluka*, was permitted. However, the restrictions on the home-coming celebrations, which were traditionally held after the boys returned from the *amabhome* in the mountains, produced some cultural trauma. The ceremony welcoming returning initiates is divided into two phases, *umphumo* and *umgidi*, which bring together local communities and families in celebration. *Umphumo* is a requirement for all initiates. However, families who have the means usually opt for *umgidi*, which is a costlier and larger celebration. Families will save long and hard to pay for this celebration, using funds in *stokvels* (local informal savings clubs) and from migrant workers, who may also contribute additional money to ensure that the *umgidi* is a high-status event which properly honours the initiates.

However, in the context of the pandemic and the new government restrictions, the vast majority of families in rural communities opted for the smaller *umphumo* celebration which is only attended by close family. This choice may have been informed by limited resources as the economy stagnated under Covid-19, as well as by concern over the rising death toll in the Eastern Cape, which brought home the lethal impacts of the virus.

During the modern initiation process, initiates are required to follow a number of steps. They must first go to a local clinic where nurses assess whether the boys are healthy, which may include testing them for Covid-19. In the company of the registered traditional surgeon (*ingcibi*) who will perform the circumcision, the boys then take the medical report to the local chief who is supposed to issue his approval for the initiation to proceed. Next, the boy goes to the police for formal approval. However, not everyone follows this same process. In some communities, boys, in response to peer pressure from their friends, go straight to the initiation school and bypass the whole medical and authorisation process. In fact, *ukuzeba*—when boys run away to join initiation schools without parental permission or the approval of nurses, chiefs or police—is quite common in these communities. In some communities no form of medical, traditional or official approval was sought by the initiates. Many people in local communities only knew about who was being initiated when they returned from the mountain. For example, parents of initiates may be so worried that their sons might die on the mountain or be bewitched that they keep the news of the initiation process within the family, only telling the broader community when they learn that the boy has healed and survived.

The South African government established the formal process of approval for initiations some time before the Covid outbreak to protect initiates, many of whom were dying as a result of botched circumcisions and unsafe treatment while on the mountain. Observance of these rules varied from area to area in the former Transkei region of the Eastern Cape. For example, in Goso, a rural community in the Ngcobo local municipality, parents decided not to allow their sons to be initiated due to fear of Covid-19, although a significant number had turned 18, the age for initiation, by the end of 2020. The decision was made even though young men who attended university faced being bullied in their new tertiary institution by older students who had gone to initiation school. One community member said: "the decision has much cost to the boys and their families, but it was a cost to take to save their lives". A parent from another rural community in the region said he had postponed the initiation plans because he was worried that if the boy tested positive for Coronavirus, which was spreading quickly, he would not gain permission to go to the mountain and would perhaps commit suicide as a result.

Initiations were also postponed on the grounds that large, crowded *umgidi* celebrations were no longer possible. These celebrations are led by the elders and attended by whole communities; traditional beer (*umqomboth*) flows freely during them. As a result, some parents decided to postpone their sons' initiations until things returned to normal, adopting a wait-and-see approach. In Qolombana, a rural location under uMhlontlo local municipality, the initiation process was postponed even though there was an initiation school in the area. Only 11 youth attended the school at the end of 2020, far short of the around 50 who usually attended, and none of these were from the village. Only one family in the district, at the nearby Sibangweni location, celebrated a coming-home ceremony for a local initiate in December 2020. In the absence of any police, few people wore masks inside the *kraal* and shared their drinks freely, as is the custom. The attendees were relaxed even though they were breaking the government's lockdown regulations. In Mhlanga rural location in Bizana, initiation schools were opened, ostensibly in adherence with the government's Covid-19 restrictions. However, some traditional leaders sought to block customary circumcisions and the opening of the schools. In one case, a young man seeking initiation had to abandon his plan to attend a local school, which had been prevented from opening, and go elsewhere.

The schools which did open their doors to initiates were supposed to follow a number of strict regulations, although they did not always comply. For example, one school flouted a rule that male circumcisions could only start from 17 December; its directors were arrested. People were arrested for breaking a number of other rules governing the operation of these schools, including the limit on 30 initiates (*abaKhwetha*) per institution; that all those involved should always wear masks; and that a proper permit for running the school had been acquired. At one institution which was operating without a permit, visiting police and health officials burnt down the school's initiation hut (*iBhoma*). However, the *abaKhwetha* were not sent home and instead a new hut was built once the police and health officials had left. In terms of overall numbers, one local police officer said there had been about 130 initiates in Bizana in December 2020, with that number perhaps rising to more than 160 when taking into account the youth who had joined without any official or parental permission. This number is much smaller than previous years. Of these initiates, more than half received *imigidi* when they came back home.

At least 15 of these initiates were hospitalised, three of whom had contracted Covid-19. In the Bizana region, most of the current generation of traditional leaders were not circumcised as youth, when initiation practices fell into abeyance. They are generally not permitted to go to the mountain to ensure the safety and health of the *abaKhwetha*, with this task thus being left to the local police. However, not all police officials wanted to go to the mountain out of fear for their own health and because of the difficulty of managing large groups of young initiates effectively.

Meanwhile, the rules about home-coming celebrations were widely flouted. Family members were told to minimise the number of people attending such celebrations, and in some areas were banned from holding even a small gathering of family members. But the restrictions did not prevent people from holding larger *imigidi* celebrations, although these were adapted to welcome home several initiates at once. For example, in one home in Bizana local municipality, there was a ceremony for two young men (*amaKrwala*). This was quite an affair and the excitement was so great that only a few people wore masks, although the *amaKrwala* themselves remembered to don them when posing for a photograph after the ceremony. The drive even in the time of Covid to hold such celebrations indicates their social and cultural importance. As well as commemorating the passage of youth to manhood, they also connect local families and communities to their ancestors. Notwithstanding the government restrictions, local people in rural areas are clearly prepared to make great efforts to perform their traditional ceremonies in acceptable and meaningful ways that are in line with their customs.[43]

In addition to male initiation rituals, performance of the *intonjane* ceremony marking a girl's passage to womanhood was also observed in rural areas of the Transkei during successive 2020 Covid-19 lockdowns. Unlike traditional male circumcision, *intonjane* takes place at various ages, from the teens to the adult years of married women and even in old age. The customs surrounding the practice can vary quite widely from community to community. Generally, the *intonjane* ceremony was subject to little government attention or regulation, in contrast with male initiation. *Intonjane* may be performed for several reasons. It may represent a cultural practice performed by every woman in a particular family at which important life lessons are imparted. Often, it is performed after a family member dreams that an ancestor is calling for the ritual. In other cases the young woman may fall sick and a *sangoma* (traditional healer) may call for the ritual to be held as a way of healing them. Historically, this ritual seemed to be performed after a girl's first period, when an older woman would warn the girl about what might happen if she has sexual relations with boys. In the modern era, *intonjane* might be delayed due to the expense of the ritual. More generally, the ritual tends to be performed in cases where the girl or woman has a particular problem that they would like to address. Older women might perform it because they cannot conceive, or because they have continual problems with their offspring. Other reasons include misfortunes in life; bed wetting; menstrual disorders; and challenges in a new marriage. A cow (which costs about R15,000) and a goat are required for the ritual. In addition, food and traditional beer (*umqombothi*) must be prepared; and certain ceremonial clothes must be provided.

One *intonjane* in a community in Zixhoseni was held as scheduled during the festive season, after all the family members had returned to the homestead from their respective places of work. During the ceremony, the girls, who were not wearing masks and had not undergone Covid-19 testing, were kept in one hut behind traditional grass mats. An open invitation was issued to people in the village to attend the ceremony; and a significant number of masked villagers accepted the invitation.[44] In the Qolombana rural location in Mhlontlo local municipality, another *intonjane* ritual, attended by six local girls, was held. Its length was cut from 30 days to only two weeks as a result of fears in relation to the pandemic. The ritual was performed because some of the girls were sick. Throughout the ceremony, there was little social distancing and no wearing of masks.[45]

The return to customary practices came with tension and uncertainty. There were several cases recorded where youth or returning urban residents differed with family elders in their interpretations of what was needed to rectify the indignity of Covid funerals or adjustments to customary practices to suit family members' travel schedules. In one case, again recorded in the Engcobo area, youth who had returned for a funeral in December were insisting that they hold the "after tears" party during the same visit, to avoid the cost of having to return in the new year. The elders firmly objected, saying that this was against tradition and would be disrespectful to the ancestors. The clash over the schedule created considerable tension, as did differing interpretations over the sequencing of rituals. The gendered and generational tensions noted in chapter five extended to the sphere of ritual. For example, young women complained that they were labelled as young wives, *makoti*, and pushed onto the front-line at funerals, attending to guests and interacting with people while others shielded themselves against infection. They felt exposed and questioned why they had to be placed at extra risk simply because they were young women.[46] The other major development was the decision of many prominent and better off rural households to host family renewal ceremonies, which often involved sacrifice, slaughtering animals and feasting, in honour of an apical family or clan ancestor. These events, which could last an entire week, were held in 2021 after the country was placed on the lowest possible level of lockdown. They appeared to represent part of a process of recentring and regeneration after the trauma of 2020.

Conclusion

On 25 January 2021, the South African MAC on Covid-19 released a memorandum stating that, following a re-evaluation of the evidence, dead Covid-19 bodies should no longer be deemed contagious. It was advised that it was only necessary for these bodies to be bagged in plastic from the hospital to the mortuary, but not thereafter. The next day, the National Funeral Practitioners Association of South Africa (Nafupa SA) met with the departments of health and home affairs and released a notice to members stating that "we are returning to the normal way of conducting funerals" and that this would "allow families to observe their cultural beliefs". Nafupa told funeral parlours there was no longer any need to triple-bag bodies in plastic, or prevent family and mourners from viewing and even touching the body, as it posed no significant health threat if appropriate precautions were taken. Nafupa members were also told that they no longer needed to deposit bodies at grave sites, but could now deliver them to the family home or churches. Coffins no longer needed to be cling-wrapped; and elaborate PPE and cleaning routines which had been being performed at the place of burial could also be abandoned. The new dispensation amounted to a massive and unexpected reversal in policy with far-reaching implications for rural communities, whose dissatisfaction with the previous policies had moved from despondency, disbelief and anger during the first wave of the pandemic to open defiance of government policy as plasticised Covid-19 bodies were illegally exhumed and reburied.

This reversal in the rules governing burial practice clearly did not come easily to the bio-medical team advising President Cyril Ramaphosa. In March 2020 the World Health Organization (WHO) had already stated that there was no evidence suggesting that Covid-19 corpses were infectious after death; this position was restated in a September 2020 WHO communique. But the MAC and the South African government had remained committed to a position which stressed the danger of dead Covid-19 bodies. The legacy and consequences of this decision have been traumatic and catastrophic for many rural African families. For these families, as well as others in the cities, the key to a successful burial is "fetching the spirit" from the place of death and safely returning it home. This requires constant communication with the spirit of the deceased. The process needs to be continuous and ongoing until the body is put in the ground. There is great danger in death for the living, which must be offset through communication with and care for the body. At home in the rural areas, the body would traditionally be viewed, engaged, washed and clothed by close relatives in the homestead overnight, and then buried the following day. The funeral service and burial rituals would usually last many hours, allowing religious leaders, family members, neighbours and traditional leaders to pay their respects and commune as they put the spirit to rest.

By comforting and calming the spirit in this way, the family would release it into the afterlife to commune with the ancestors. However, the regulations introduced around bagging the body and delivering it directly to the grave site; cling-wrapping coffins; and fumigating houses and grave sites created enormous spiritual anxiety and popular anger. Traditional leaders largely ignored these feelings during the first wave, strongly supporting the Covid-19 regulations published under the Disaster Management Act. The metaphor used in rural communities across the Eastern Cape to describe the government's approach was *ukuvala isango* or "closing the gate", which referred to a process of rural people being shut out by government, even from their own cultural practices.

CONCLUSION

POST-COVID RESET

Nostalgia

When the Iron Curtain was removed across Europe in 1991, many families left Eastern Europe for Western Europe because they wanted to escape the memory of communism and embrace liberal modernity and capitalism in the West.[1] In countries such as Hungary an entire generation of young people left for jobs and a new life in Western cities.[2] Similar migration happened in the rural peripheries of South Africa as apartheid came to an end. Five years after the introduction of democracy in 1994, the former ethnic homelands were emptying as youth and women flooded to the cities with new expectations of freedom and modernity. They hoped for employment and a better life which would come with the promised urban transformation, universal service delivery, free housing for the poor and an anticipated economic boom.[3] The idea swept through the rural areas that "life is everywhere": all you had to do was leave and get it. There was hope for a transformed form of capitalism, which would be inclusive, non-racial and developmental. This would build a new society in which suburban life, affluence and democratic citizenship would be accessible to everyone who left the rural areas and came to the city. Youth and women in the rural areas, who had been prevented from accessing the city and joining the pool of urban labour under apartheid, yearned to participate in the fruits of democracy and the benefits of freedom. However, the problem for South Africa was even greater than the challenges faced in Europe at the end of the Cold War. The "promised land"—the big cities of Johannesburg, Durban and Cape Town—had neither the homes nor the jobs that the new mobile population desired.[4] There were no dedicated reception areas for migrants, nor any desire to release land for the urbanising masses. They were forced into informal settlements and township backyards, and charged relatively high rents while they eked out a precarious living in the new burgeoning informal sector, as they waited for proper jobs and houses.[5] In general, the ANC's promise of residential security and stable employment as a foundation of future suburban bliss never materialised. By comparison, the prospects for Eastern European migrants with skills and an education were generally better. They often found jobs and secured decent places to live in the old cities of Western Europe, while remitting surplus income to their families back home, in countries which were struggling to adjust to the new normal of capitalist restructuring.[6]

In post-Soviet Eastern Europe, the belief that affluence, freedom and prosperity would come easily after the arrival of democracy and capitalism was widely embraced, even though there was no evidence to suggest that the "normalcy of liberalism" would ever be achieved in this region.[7] The dawning realisation that the "light of liberalism" was not as bright as had been expected and was failing to deliver a new modernity brought disillusion and populist politics to the region. The inequalities and arrogance of the new consultant-driven, externally led, neo-liberal form of capitalism alienated local people. They began to re-engage with ideas of nationalism and pre-socialist nativism, arguing that survival in troubled times would not be achieved through the promise of individualism and cosmopolitanism, but needed to be renegotiated through the strength of local cultures, collective effort and allegiance to the old nation. Eastern European populist leaders declared that they remained pure and true to a Europe that had not yet been diluted and contaminated by unnecessary immigration and assimilation, unlike their Western European counterparts, who were inviting immigrants to flood across their borders. They argued that those who bowed to the winds of liberalism and cosmopolitanism had lost their identity.[8]

In his 2015 book, *Democracy as Death: The Moral Order of Anti-liberal Politics in South Africa*, Jason Hickel found that a "men of two worlds" ideology remained strong among Zulu-speaking migrant workers in the sugar mills and factories of Durban and surrounding towns in Kwa-Natal. These men rejected democracy and the ANC.[9] One worker from Kwa-Mashu in Durban said: "there is a problem with democracy, it has become like a curse in the ears of the ancestors and can bring about misfortune that can lead to death."[10] Another worker, interviewed in 2009, said that the ANC had "turned everything upside down [and] because of democracy, now the women and the men are becoming the same, the ancestors are displeased, and many misfortunes are coming on us". These mainly middle-aged migrant men expressed antipathy towards democracy, gender equality and the lack of moral authority, discipline, and social order in the city. They still spoke in a language of sharp urban and rural contrasts, rejecting the modernising influences of the ruling ANC, which they accused of idealising morally degraded and chaotic city life. For these men, the true African heart of the country still lay in the local countryside, where the social order of Zulu homesteads provided a patriarchal script for the reconstruction of the nation. This need for moral restoration and a rejection of neo-liberalism was expressed before the Marikana massacre in August 2011, when dozens of miners were shot dead, many in their backs, by the South African police in the hills around the platinum mines. The striking miners had withdrawn from mine premises and taken refuge in the hills (*koppies*) to regroup and wait for a settlement. In the days before the massacre, the "mountain committee" was led by Xhosa-speaking migrants from the Eastern Cape.[11] This grouping spoke of the need to restore the values of the "old nation" and embrace the wisdom of the *amadoda* (senior miners and men). They employed an Mpondo traditional healer and his sons to help prepare the miners for an impending war with the mine bosses and ANC-aligned National Miner Workers Union (MWU). Not all the striking workers bought into this narrative, but a significant portion paid towards bringing the healer onto the mountain to dose the workers with war medicines and animal fat in preparation for battle.[12]

In her 2020 book, *Nostalgia after Apartheid: Disillusion, Youth and Democracy in South Africa*, Amber Reed notes that she discovered high levels of disillusionment with South Africa's democratic transition among rural youth and older people in a small rural town in the Transkei.[13] Her fieldwork highlighted local nostalgia for a more orderly, morally upright rural lifestyle which, in memory, offered greater opportunities for youth employment. There was a yearning for the agrarian ethos of the 20th century Transkei. Reed notes that, while many youths felt bored, disempowered, and excluded, many in the older generation complained that there was no longer any respect, decency or neighbourly cooperation in the village. The old folk lamented rising rates of rural crime; a low level of interest in agricultural production; and the absence of village-based social cohesion, as well as a general loss of respect for and adherence to the values of "Xhosa culture". Many seemed to feel that something valuable had been lost which needed to be restored. There was a palpable nostalgia for a time of greater social cohesion and a stronger commitment to local economic and social development. Many of the older generation said there had been more respect and dignity in rural life under the Transkei government of Kaiser Matanzima, the apartheid era homeland strongman.[14]

This sense of disillusionment was expressed during the 2021 local government elections, where rural voter turnout dropped off dramatically. One report from November 2021 noted that rural residents in the Transkei even locked polling stations to stop people from voting for the ruling party. Journalist Mkhuseli Sizani, from the not-for-profit news agency *Ground Up*, reported one extreme case where:

> On election day, the villagers of Phungulelweni shut down the voting station in Ward 13 of Ntabankulu Local Municipality. They padlocked Phungulelweni Junior Primary School in protest over a lack of water and bad roads. Voter turnout dropped from 55% in 2016 to 2% in 2021, with only nine voters and 18 ballots cast. There are 420 households in the area and 433 registered voters. Ironically, the handful of votes for the ANC (with 16 votes and two votes going to the Economic Freedom Fighters) gave the party a slightly higher percentage of the vote (89%) than in 2016. Overall, in the ward the ANC got 84%.

> According to residents, police were called to cut off the padlocks, but people still did not turn up to vote. "I am 70 years old and it is the first time in my life seeing our people fed up with the ANC," said Mavalela

Ntlukaniso, a village headman. "Voting used to be so exciting here." But a lack of service delivery and empty promises angered the community. "We believe the decision we took should teach all the officials, especially those who belong to the ANC, to respect the voters."[15]

This article does not mention a factor which is clear from the contents of this book and interviews after the election: the negative impact that the state's management of the Covid pandemic had on voter support for the ruling party, which for the first time in 27 years registered less than 50% of the 30% of eligible voters that cast their ballot on 1 November 2021.[16]

Ritual and double-rootedness

In their work on ritual and social change, economic anthropologists Stephen Gudeman and Chris Hann have argued that ritual played a critical role in re-anchoring families and communities in Eastern Europe as the socialist state collapsed and their lives were turned upside down by the shock therapy of neo-liberalism.[17] In this context, they argue, rural residents returned to kin-based modes of trust and cooperation—the community social economy, or what Gudeman calls "the base"[18]—by dismantling the socialist collectives and placing the family or household at the centre of rural social and economic life, as had been the case prior to the 1950s.[19] This return to the base did not reconstruct the pre-socialist peasantry, but rebuilt the human economy based on a kinship that focused on producing new kinds of rural livelihoods. Gudeman and Hann highlight the role played by family ritual in recreating or restoring relations *within* and especially *among* households in broken rural communities.[20] Without the safety net of the socialist system, families were caught up in a dis-embedded market economy that individualised their plight in the absence of the socialist ethos of government-led community building and state loyalty. Under socialism, ritual was extensively used by the state to encourage social cohesion, especially when the system of collective provisioning failed to meet local needs—for example, when production targets were not met due to resistance on collective farms.[21] To offset local grievances produced by production failures, special days, ritual and festivals were created by the state to redistribute resources and entertain families, while also fostering political loyalty to the state. After socialism, these government-invented ritual events fell away and pre-socialist religious, family and community traditions returned, reconnecting families to an older set of values, identities, and social practices.[22]

These changes in the ritual and festival calendar and the regearing of the social economy for survival under post-socialist conditions informed the subsequent rise of populism and nationalism. They also provided the context for youth dissatisfaction, and the large scale migration away from the rural areas for Western cities. Many rural young people did not want to reconstruct their lives from the shards of pre-socialist rural values, which they felt were unfit to support long-term survival in the new world. At the same time, the reconstruction of family values and nationalism also touched this generation profoundly; leaders like Orbán in Hungary appealed to the youth not to forget their "homeland". The ambivalence of the youth to the new "homeland" traditions that were being forged may also indicate the dual or fluid role played by ritual in both supporting and disrupting established systems of social value.[23] In this regard, Gudeman and Hann conclude that the new rituals did not always reinforce old values. They also helped communities to break with the past and build new kinds of social relations:

> For us rituals are related to economy by the social connections they *make or break*. Rituals express, reiterate and sustain social ties. They make and recognise relations to others, but they can sever them, as in the case of rites of passage. Rituals are often essential in extending sociality, as in gestures of friendliness, hospitality and words of kindness; they can connect, or disguise and even mystify social relations.[24]

This volume has explored the centrality of ritual in the making and remaking of a former South African homeland, which was also previously a colonial labour reserve. It has described how rural African communities restructured themselves at the turn of the 20th century as they lost their political sovereignty, autonomy, and access to land. Under colonial rule, local people's focus shifted away from pastoralism, which required large amounts of land, to more intensive agrarianism. This helped them retain a measure of social and economic independence. Constrained access to land was reinforced by the 1913 Land Act after Union in South Africa. At this time, new neighbourhood rituals were created which encouraged and activated relationships among households, leveraging the technical advancements in colonial agriculture to help rural communities refocus their livelihoods. The adjusted and innovative cultural system embraced the imperative towards permanent settlement but also necessitated migrant labour. The land could not sustain families and communities, who also had to pay colonial taxes. In this process, a neighbourhood and regional moral economy based on age and gender hierarchies was reconstructed. The focus during this period was on building an agrarian ethos, which protected access to land and created strong territorial identities. Ritual was critical to this process and helped to clearly distinguish the countryside from the city.[25] The rural "homeland" was positioned as a place of agrarian production and bucolic bliss, and underpinned the emergence of a powerful set of morally and politically charged oppositions between the "goodness" of rurality and the cultural and moral "degradation" of the city. From the 1950s, apartheid restructuring and forced resettlement in the ethnic homelands cut away at the agrarianism, but not at the fictions or consciousness of migrants that South Africa was comprised of different kinds of places.

The argument of this book is that this opposition, which is now being restored in places with the rise of populism and the politics of nostalgia, started to dissolve after apartheid and reintegration of the homelands into common South Africa. The ANC's policies favoured urbanisation and ended institutionalised systems of population control and enforced labour migration. One of the first targets of the ANC's Reconstruction and Development Programme (RDP) in housing was the transformation of single-sex municipal hostels across the country into family housing units. Indeed, the entire focus of the RDP was on offering suburban homes, basic services and living conditions to poor families on the fringes of the cities. The ANC now claims to have delivered well over 3 million homes to poor people in towns and cities over the past 27 years. For most of that period, the housing subsidy scheme was not offered in rural areas, although basic services such as access to electricity, communal taps and improved roads and infrastructure were meant to be delivered to improve rural lives. The problem for those who urbanised was that there were very few decent formal jobs in the cities that paid enough to allow them to transform their RDP starter homes into fully-fledged suburban homes. There were also too many rural relatives arriving in the cities for them to keep their sites free of backyard shacks and rent to supplement their urban incomes. Many RDP housing estates, especially those that were well positioned relative to urban jobs, were thus informally re-urbanised. New shack areas were also full of small younger households who urbanised without jobs and waited for access to the urban housing lists.

But none of this substantially diminished the desire amongst the urbanising poor and working classes to retain a rural base in the countryside. The inclination towards double-rootedness was strengthened when the ANC offered social grants and pensions to help rural families cope with poverty, giving them a sense of dignity and independence that had been lacking when they depended entirely on irregular migrant remittances. In this context the sub-urban nationalism promoted by the ruling party in the cities was displaced to the rural areas, where households had access to land for new housing and could make their own building blocks, as well as buy building materials from the hardware stores in towns. With the same supermarkets and DIY chain stores now traversing the country, purchases could be made in the city and delivered in the countryside. In addition, the desire to rebuild the homestead in rural areas was profoundly impacted by the AIDS pandemic which took hundreds of thousands of lives and brought premature death and suffering. Those who were fatally sick in the cities often returned home, or were taken home in coffins once they had passed away in the cities. This stimulated the growth of a post-apartheid funeral and death insurance industry in the cities, but also recalibrated doubled-rootedness, intensifying the movement of people and bodies across space. Drawing on their insurance policies and pooled family resources, rural funerals became an opportunity for families to pull together. They could demonstrate resilience and perform upward social mobility by hosting lavish funerals, often funded by debt,[26] as they enhanced their claims to suburban style modernity and the new forms of citizenship encouraged by the state.

CONCLUSION

Rupture and reconnection

By the time Covid hit, the cost of rural funerals had skyrocketed to well over a third of the total annual income of families in most parts of the country. The services offered by urban entrepreneurs in the death industry were diverse and seemingly endless; attending or planning for funerals was a major business. Planning for death and burials in the countryside had become something of an obsession in township and informal settlements; there was constant family networking and talk of investing or saving for rural homebuilding or death, especially amongst women. Social media was full of stories and pictures, posted by urban women, of improved rural homes. Mentioning personal agency in the realisation of such achievements ran the risk of envy, so the work completed was invariably attributed to the "Grace of God", the profits from informal savings groups or the generosity of family. Although travelling between town and countryside for leisure and long holidays was not as frequent as in the past, it was difficult for close family members to not return home for funerals because these rituals were based on pooled resources and expressed family unity and identity. In this book we have shown how rural funerals were gradually transformed after apartheid from modest neighbourhood events to large village affairs, with taxi loads of mourners arriving for the weekend from the cities. In the past, the aim was to bury the dead quickly and start the long period of mourning. A celebration of the life of the deceased occurred at the end of this period, with additional rituals and the scattering of clothes and possessions around the homestead.

With the post-apartheid period of urbanisation, the AIDS pandemic and the rise of the funeral industry, burial was often suspended for weeks as the body was put on ice to allow all the families arrangements to be concluded and plans for the rural return finalised. The extension of the time between death and burial added to the costs because it gave families time to discuss the appropriate send-off at home. Many of those we interviewed said that the rise in costs happened almost invisibly as each item, from the tombstone to the transport to the catering, was discussed and debated within the family. As one veteran of several recent family funerals explained: "you hardly notice it when it is happening, but the costs just rise, and in the end the bill is a massive hang-over that lingers for years".[27] He added that: "getting the house right so that I could project a good view of the family was also a key part of this too". But the trend towards large and expensive funerals also occurred in the rural areas, especially as traditional leaders and rural clerics saw these events as opportunities to legitimise their roles. In the cases presented, for example, we saw how in 2019 Zipho went to the traditional leaders to ask for a rapid funeral for her mother but was persuaded to put her body on ice till the end of the month, to allow urban family to book leave and arrange transport. All the while, Zipho had to feed a group of live-in mourners and funeral helpers. At the funeral, traditional leaders spoke at length to endorse the family and the deceased as valued community members in front of a large audience. The more taxis that came from the cities the better.[28] Some clerics and churches used funerals as opportunities to evangelise. Against a background of widespread rural poverty, funerals were pinnacles of family self-representation. The causes of death remained public secrets while the secrets of private, family life were made public. Indeed, as Potelwa remarked, the funerals became like the "after tears" events that happened after mourning, when the focus was on celebrating the deceased and the family rather than mourning the dead.[29]

By April 2020, the fluid and interconnected urban and rural social economy of death, consolidated and reenforced by the (sub)urbanisation of the countryside, came to an end. Lockdown was announced and travel between provinces was banned and criminalised. There was also simultaneously a massive clampdown on customary practices and large rural funerals, which were shut down by force. It was no longer possible for huge groups of urban relatives and friends to return home for a long weekend. In chapter three, we illustrated the extent and nature of the clampdown, which occurred at short notice and with little communication about the new rules and procedures to rural families. Shortly after lockdown there was a limited window for reverse migration around Easter, after which movement was shut down as the police swarmed through the countryside closing initiation schools and overturning pots of beer and meat at funeral gatherings.

The police were given a central role in the management of death under Covid. They were empowered to issue death certificates and had to authorise and monitor funerals. They were charged with the responsibility of ensuring that the Disaster Management Act was enforced in rural areas, and that social distancing was observed, rules followed, registers kept and sanitisers used. The state regulations also did not tolerate any delays between death and burial. In mid-2020, when Covid deaths rose sharply across the country, burial was required five days after death. Bodies were wrapped in plastic and only one or two family members were allowed to view the corpse at a time at the mortuary. The delivery of the dead to the rural burial site only occurred on the day of the funeral, and coffins were taken directly to the graves, which were sometimes closed-up before the mourners had arrived there from the main house. Many of these procedures were implemented for the state by the funeral parlours, who had to comply with strict government regulations to retain their licences. Funeral parlour staff that travelled with the coffins wore safety hazmat suits and moved around with spray tanks of sanitiser on their backs. The world of death and burial rituals was turned upside down.

By the end of the year, communities and families were so trauma-tised that they started to boycott funerals and only gathered in num-bers for "after tears" parties held a week or so after the death. The absence of kin, neighbours and relatives from the funerals under-mined the legitimacy of death rituals; an empty funeral tent was normally a sign of an unworthy life and a lack of endorsement of the family by the community. The spirits of people buried in this manner could easily wander and their safe passage to the afterlife was far from secure. The reluctance of neighbours and relatives to attend these funerals was, however, driven by fear rather than disapproval. This fear was created by the state's enforcement of the law and the President's encouragement of rural people to stay away and defer their family rituals. It was not just the cultivation of fear that instilled spiritual insecurity, but also the way bodies were managed and treated: they were cut off from communication with the living, wrapped and bound in plastic (tossed aside like "trash" in the ground) and covered with dirt before relatives could say their final goodbyes. Our book has documented these processes in detail and illustrated not only how dignity was lost as rural culture was blamed for the pandemic, causing people doubt and distress, but also how the very possibilities of social reproduction at the margins were cut away. Indeed, social reproduction is never simply a process of biological reproduction, catered for by a social grant, but always involves the creation and reproduction of identities, networks and the mutuality need to make life possible.[30] As a result, it is not surprising that, once the lockdown restrictions were lifted, families took matters into their own hands by exhuming and reburying the dead. After a deadly second wave hit at the end of 2020, families started to plan reunions that reaffirmed their connection to their home and the land of their ancestors. With the reopening of initiation lodges and the re-establishing of customary practices late in 2020, people defiantly rejected the rules and precautions that had been imposed on them. They expressed a spirit of resistance and open disregard for rules of a state that had "closed the gate" on them and disrespected their way of life and beliefs.

In addition to revealing the transformations of funerals and family rituals in the time of Covid, this book has also exposed the absence of productive engagement between ordinary people and the state, as a bio-medical fix to the global health crisis was pursued. The chapter on gatekeepers and go-betweens illustrates that chiefs and traditional leaders feared infection and often stayed away from the sites of death and burial, while clerics and spiritual leaders remained more committed to ensuring that there could still be dignity in death and smooth passage to the afterlife. The police and nurses were widely criticised for their arrogance and disregard for the plight of the poor and suffering. We argue that this distance was not new but a product of a pre-existing top-down and authoritarian bureaucratic culture in the rural areas, created under apartheid and extended after democracy. Many who worked for the homeland civil service in the Transkei retained their jobs after liberation and worked in the police stations and clinics after democracy. This was reflected in the belief that local bureaucrats remained arrogant and indifferent to suffering. We further argue that these attitudes and orientations stymied the rise of a "people's science", like the response in West Africa to Ebola of the 2010s. They also prevented the co-production of preventative strategies at the community level, in collaboration with health employees, government officials and community leaders. The exclusion of the traditional healers from the conversation about Covid was symptomatic of the larger problem. During the first wave, the collapse and closure of government departments and public health facilities was a striking feature of the unfolding crisis and the rural poor's experience of the gate closing in the former homelands.[31] Civil servants and nurses shut facilities because they feared for their lives and were not prepared to operate in the absence of adequate personal protective equipment or the availability of deep cleaning services to reopen clinics, hospitals, and government offices.

Post-Covid rural reset

We started this book by contending that, by declaring national "war on Covid" through the passage of the Disaster Management Act in March 2020 and enforcing that law across the country, the state created what the Italian philosopher Gorgio Agamben has called a "state of exception". The individual rights of citizens were suspended to allow the state to wage war against the Covid pathogen. In considering the narratives, discourses and practices of the state during the Covid lockdown during 2020, we arrived at the conclusion that the South African state did not regard all citizens as equal. Following Friedman's argument in *One Virus, Two Nations*, we suggested that the state adopted different strategies for the management of Covid in rich and poor areas, and also imposed a greater state of exception on rural populations in the former homelands. The latter were not just seen as less capable of self-regulating and individualising their behaviours than middle-class suburbanites, but were said to be bearers of cultural traits and forms of mutuality (*ubuntu*) that carried special danger for the spread of the virus. These places were also known to have weak bio-medical and public health systems that would collapse with widespread infection, as seen in chapter two. This assessment of the special conditions in these areas resulted in the unfolding of forms of repression and control that were excessive and inhuman, and allowed the state to violate people's cultural rights, dignity and sense of spiritual security in unacceptable ways. Indeed, by targeting rituals and customary practices without property consulting rural people, explaining the nature of the threat or involving them in solutions, the state intensified social divides between people and the state, youth and elders, men and women and traditional healers and health officials. The great irony and bitter twist in this tale is that, when a Covid tsunami returned to the Eastern Cape in the final months of 2020 for a second wave, it caught the urban bureaucrats with co-morbidities in the Buffalo City with devastating force. In December 2020 and January 2021, the death rate in the regional capital of Buffalo City, where the middle classes still had money to celebrate Christmas, exceeded 350 people per 100,000.[32]

This schism between rural elites—including nurses, police, bureaucrats and many traditional leaders—and ordinary people has been highlighted at various point in the book. The idea that national elites and bio-medical scientists tried to tightly control the management of the pandemic from the centre is without dispute, but it is also true that many of their instructions were filtered down through provincial and district level command councils, creating other layers of involvement and calibration. We have specifically highlighted the role of gatekeepers, and how politicians at the regional level, as well as traditional leaders, implemented the instructions they received from the National Command Council—sometimes against their own interests. This compounded the confusion and crisis in rural areas. As a former homeland, the Transkei area had been controlled from the centre, through patronage politics, long before the ANC came to power. Bureaucrats there understood what was at stake if they did not follow orders from above. This dynamic was particularly evident in the field of public health, where the provincial minister and her team were lambasted for their incompetent response to priming the regional health system into high alert in April 2020. The provincial minister was publicly shamed and scolded, then blamed for rising infections in urban and rural areas. The focus on control rather than prevention and protection was, however, only part of the reason that the local healthcare systems collapsed so quickly from the moment infections rose, as seen in chapter three.

But the critical weaknesses in the provincial public health system and its failure to do its core business were already well-known a decade earlier, fully exposed in the cutting, comprehensive and widely publicised 2013 report by NGOs and doctors entitled: *Death and Dying in the Eastern Cape: An Investigation into the Collapse of a Health System*. Rural clinics were essentially pill collection centres and were mostly out of drugs long before Covid struck. The hospitals were hopelessly understaffed, physically crumbling and poorly equipped. Indeed, it appears that the state abandoned the idea of shoring up this broken and dysfunctional bio-medical system from the outset and focused only on what could be done at a handful of urban hospitals, especially the Livingstone Hospital in Nelson Mandela Bay, which became the focus of global media reports in July 2020. The state's promises of sending Covid trained nurses to rural clinics and additional support to rural hospitals never materialised, resulting in strikes and walk-outs. The approach of the state in the rural areas was thus not calibrated for the realities in rural areas, and was sinister and dishonest in its awareness of the challenges in the public health system.

In June 2021, the award-winning Eastern Cape health journalist Estelle Ellis wrote an article called "Death and dying in the Eastern Cape continued: what to do when losing hope is not an option", where she suggests that "public hospitals have become a place befitting a quote from the Italian poet and writer Dante Alighieri's *Inferno*: "Abandon All Hope, Ye Who Enter Here". She goes on to wonder:

> Perhaps this will be a moment when civil societies, communities, religious leaders and businesses join hands and say: No more.... Perhaps after decades of hobbling along, critically wounded, the Eastern Cape health department, relying on the resilience of its doctors and nurses, can finally become a new model for what public health should look like. Perhaps the chance is now as the mighty bureaucrats are in a weakened state. Perhaps now is the time to invite hope to return. Nobody else is coming for the Eastern Cape. The province will have to save itself.[33]

The absence of any community-based, preventative healthcare strategies in the face of the pandemic has left a legacy, seen not only at the polls in the 2021 elections but also in the high rates of vaccine hesitancy and resistance. The government is struggling to increase vaccine uptake in rural areas, despite a much stronger rural outreach strategy with NGO and private sector support. People in rural areas are suspicious of the state's intentions and all manner of stories have circulated concerning the content and impact of the vaccines. This aspect of the crisis is part of an ongoing enquiry that we are currently working on. However, when drawing attention to the public health systems failures of rural communities, we have consistently referred to the experience in West African countries during the Ebola outbreaks of the early 2010s. In the absence of strong rural health system, anthropologists, doctors and NGOs like Médecins Sans Frontières (MSF) brought bio-medical experts and communities together to co-produce preventative strategies at the local level that made sense culturally, socially and bio-medically. Richards calls this process of practical knowledge creation a "people's science" because it seeks to devise preventative strategies and actions that minimise infection and maximise care and participation, by working with and through local knowledge systems and everyday social practices. In South Africa, there has recently been a dearth of similar strategies, despite the long-term involvement of MSF and other NGOS in some rural areas.[34] As Ellis suggests, considerable energy, effort and resources should be focused on this area as the pandemic lingers and disaffection with the state and the public health system deepens.

This brings us finally to the role of ritual in the making and remaking of the human economy of migrant labour. The national campaign to vaccinate rural populations is gaining momentum in South Africa with new players, including NGOs like Right to Care, assisting the state with the distribution of vaccines in rural areas. It is clearly unlikely that the fear and terror of 2020 will return to these areas again in the time of the Covid pandemic, certainly not in the way it has been described above. This is already evident from interviews conducted in late 2021, where local people state that communities had largely internalised the threat of the pandemic but certainly not forgotten the way in which they were treated. This is evident in their response to the ruling party during the November 2021 elections. The big question that remains now is how the systems of trans-locality and double-rootedness, which have been prominent in these areas in the past century, will adapt and change, and be reconstituted and remade after Covid. Will there be a recovery and reinvention of ritual and customary practice that can sustain the levels of rural and urban interconnections seen in the past three decades, underpinned by urban unemployment, the AIDS pandemic and the rise of the funeral industry? Will families cut back on the large investment they made in rural rituals, especially family funerals and rural house building, and return to more modest forms of rural homemaking? Can this be achieved with new low-carbon technologies and off-the-grid self-reliance? Will the possibility of a Basic Income Grant (BIG) provide support for the urban transition that the ruling party has sought, but failed to realise; or will there be a greater tendency towards rural return and reverse migration as the economic crisis of consumer capitalism deepens in South Africa? Given the current levels of dissatisfaction in rural areas, are we on the cusp of widespread rural revolts like those seen in the 1950s and early 1960s, when rural Transkei exploded in protest with apartheid restructuring? Will there finally be a set of policies in the South African state that recognise the complex interconnection between town and country, trans-locality and legacies of migrant labour, and not just talk of separate systems of urban versus rural development? Is it possible that neighbourliness will again replace family pride as the basis of rural mutuality to stimulate a return to rural agrarianism and production?

There is some evidence now, especially with the vaccination programme, that health officials are starting to reach out to rural communities in more meaningful ways. However, these initiatives cannot be analysed in isolation from the larger social and economic questions regarding the impact of Covid on rural poverty and the future dynamics of the culture of migration.

APPENDICES

Appendix 1: Regulations governing funerals and the treatment of the deceased produced by the South African government and the World Health Organization

Attendance of funerals

35. (1) Movement between provinces, metropolitan areas or districts by a person intending to attend a funeral is only permitted if the person is a
    (a) spouse or partner of the deceased;
    (b) child or grandchild of the deceased, whether biological, adopted. stepchild, or a foster child;
    (c) child-in-law of the deceased;
    (d) parent of the deceased, whether biological, adopted or stepparent;
    (e) sibling, whether biological, adopted or stepbrother or sister of the deceased; or
    (f) grandparent of the deceased;
    (2) Attendance at a funeral is limited to 50 persons and is not regarded as a prohibited gathering.
    (3) Night vigils are prohibited.
    (4) During a funeral, all health protocols and social distancing measures must be adhered to in order to limit exposure of persons at the funeral to COVID-19.

(5) Each person, whether travelling alone or not, wishing to attend a funeral and who has to travel between metropolitan areas, districts, or between provinces, must obtain a permit which corresponds substantially with Form 4 of Annexure A, from his or her nearest magistrate's office or police station to travel to the funeral and back.

(6) The head of court, or a person designated by him or her, or a station commander of a police station or a person designated by him or her, may issue the permit to travel to a funeral.

(7) Upon a request for a permit to attend a funeral, a person requesting a permit must produce a death certificate or a certified copy of the death certificate to the head of court, or a person designated by him or her, or a station commander of a police station or a person designated by him or her: Provided that where a death certificate is not yet available, and the funeral must be held within 24 hours in keeping with cultural or religious practices, the person requesting the permit must make a sworn affidavit which corresponds with Form 5 of Annexure A, together with a letter from a cultural or religious leader confirming the need for the funeral to take place within 24 hours.

(8) Only two family members of the deceased may, with the required permits, travel in the vehicle transporting the mortal remains to the metropolitan area, district, or province where the funeral will take place if the cause of death of the deceased being transported is non-COVID-19 related: Provided that the health protocols and social distancing measures are adhered to.

(9) The provisions of regulation 43 must be strictly adhered to when travelling.

(10) A copy of the permit issued and the death certificate or sworn affidavit made, must be kept safely by the head of court, or station commander of a police station, for record keeping for a period of three months after the national state of disaster has ended, whereafter it may be destroyed.

(11) All forms must be completed in full, including full names, identification or passport numbers and full contact details as required in the form.

(12) A form that is not completed in full as required by sub-regulation (11) is invalid.

Appendix 2: *Extract from Department of Health. 2020. Amendment to the directions issued in terms of regulation 10(1) of the regulations made under section 27(2) of the Disaster Management Act, 2002: Measures to address, prevent and combat the spread of Covid-19. 25 May.*

Handling of mortal remains: General

8A (1) The handling, transportation, importation, exportation and final disposal of COVID-19 mortal remains should be conducted only in accordance with Chapters 4, 5 and 6 of the Human Remains Regulations.

(2) All persons handling COVID-19 mortal remains should wear suitable personal protective clothing at all times.

(3) All persons handling COVID-19 mortal remains should practise good personal hygiene such as washing hands with soap and water and using personal protective clothing.

(4) No person may at any given time make contact with, or touch, the mortal remains without wearing the appropriate PPE.

(5) Metropolitan and local municipalities should ensure that the burial or cremation of COVID-19 mortal remains takes place in suitably approved cemeteries or crematoria, respectively.

(6) Metropolitan and district municipalities should ensure that they identify areas that may be utilised for mass burial should the need for same arise.

Handling of mortal remains in mortuaries or at funeral undertakers

8B. (1) The act of moving a recently deceased patient onto a hospital trolley for transportation to the mortuary might be sufficient to expel small amounts of air from the lungs and thereby present a minor risk.

(2) A body bag should be used for transferring the body to the mortuary and those handling the body at this point should use full PPE.

(3) The outer surface of the body bag should be decontaminated immediately before the body bag leaves the ward or anteroom area and may require at least two individuals wearing such protective clothing, in order to manage this process.

(4) The trolley carrying the body must be disinfected prior to leaving the ward or anteroom.

(5) Prior to leaving the ward or anteroom, the staff members must remove their PPE.

(6) Once in the hospital or private mortuary, it would be acceptable to open the body bag for family viewing by family members (one at a time) only at the mortuary. Family must be provided with masks and gloves for the viewing and should not touch the body with bare hands. Mortuary attendant must wear full PPE.

(7) Washing or preparing of the mortal remains is allowed provided those carrying out the task wear PPE such as gloves, masks and waterproof coverall, and all PPEs used must be disposed of immediately. However, the washing and preparing of the mortal remains by family members is not encouraged due to the health risks.

(8) Mortuary staff and funeral directors must be advised by the Environmental Health Practitioner of the biohazard risk.

(9) No washing is allowed out of the mortuary or funeral undertaker's premises.

(10) If the family wishes to dress the body, they may do so at the funeral undertaker's premises prior to the body being placed in the body bag and those carrying out the task should wear PPE such as gloves, masks and waterproof coverall aprons, and all PPEs used must be disposed of immediately.

(11) If a post-mortem is required, safe working techniques should be used and full PPE should be worn.

(12) In order to avoid excessive manipulation of the body, embalming is not recommended, however, if embalming is undertaken, the embalmer should wear full PPE.

(13) After use, empty body bags should be cut and disposed of as health care risk waste.

(14) After use, the reusable empty heavy-duty body bags must be treated in terms of existing procedures.

Measures when a person passes on at home

8C. (1) In the event that a person infected with COVID-19 dies at home, family members must not, at any stage, handle the body. An EMS [emergency medical service] must be called immediately to confirm death before removal by an undertaker.

(2) The belongings of the deceased person should be handled with gloves and cleaned with a detergent followed by disinfection with a solution of at least 70% ethanol or 0.1% (1000 ppm) bleach.

(3) Clothing and other fabric belongings of the deceased should be machine washed with warm water and laundry detergent at 60–90 °C (140–194 °F).

(4) If machine washing is not possible, linens can be soaked in hot water and soap in a large drum using a stick to stir and being careful to avoid splashing.

(5) The drum should then be emptied, and the linens soaked in 0.05% chlorine for approximately 30 minutes. Finally, the laundry should be rinsed with clean water and the linens should be allowed to dry in full sunlight.

Conveyance of infectious mortal remains

8D. (1) The mortal remains of a COVID-19 patient may not be conveyed in public in any way unless:

    (a) such remains are placed in a polythene bag, sealed in an airtight container, placed in a sturdy non-transparent sealed coffin, embalmed and the total surface of the body is covered with a 5cm layer of wood sawdust or other absorbent material which is treated with a disinfectant;

(b) a medical practitioner declares, in writing, that in his or her opinion the conveyance of such mortal remains will not constitute a health hazard: and

(c) the body is transported in an authorised vehicle designated and certified to transport mortal remains.

(2) No person other than an attending medical practitioner, an attending forensic pathologist or a medical practitioner who can prove that he or she has treated the deceased during illness, may certify that the person did not die of an infectious disease. A certificate or declaration that a person did not die of an infectious disease must:

(a) accompany the mortal remains at all times during the conveyance and up to the burial; and

(b) be shown to an Environmental Health Practitioner on demand, by the person responsible for the conveyance of the mortal remains.

(3) No person may:

(a) damage a polythene bag or a sturdy non-transparent sealed coffin;

(b) open such bag or coffin;

(c) remove the mortal remains from the bag or coffin; or

(d) come into direct contact with the mortal remains after the bag or coffin has been sealed.

Prohibition of viewing and storage of body at home

8E. A funeral undertaker must deliver the mortal remains on the morning of burial, and not the night before the burial, and must ensure that the remains are not touched during viewing.

Environmental cleaning and control

8F. (1) The mortuary must be kept clean and properly ventilated and illuminated at all times.

(2) Surfaces and instruments should be made of materials that can be easily disinfected as prescribed in the Human Remains Regulations.

(3) Surfaces, where the body was prepared, should first be cleaned with soap and water, or a commercially prepared detergent solution. After cleaning, a disinfectant with a minimum concentration of 0.1% (1000 ppm) sodium hypochlorite (bleach) or 70% ethanol should be used to disinfect.

Disposal of mortal remains: Burial or cremation

8G. (1) Cremation is highly recommended where a person has passed on due to COVID-19.

(2) A burial or cremation of the mortal remains of a person who died of COVID-19 must be carried out in terms of the Human Remains Regulations.

(3) (a) Burial services should be as short as possible but may not exceed two hours in order to minimise possible exposure.

(b) Mourners should observe physical distancing during and after the burial service.

(4) Only close family members should attend a funeral service of a person that died of COVID-19 or of other infectious diseases.

(5) For the purposes of protecting the health of the mourners at a burial service, a COVID-19 patient should not attend a burial service irrespective of his or her relationship with the deceased.

(6) Those tasked with placing the body in the grave, on the funeral pyre, etc. should wear gloves and wash hands with soap and water once the burial is complete.

Disposal of Mortal Remains in High-Risk Situation

8H. (a) The mortal remains may not be kept for more than three days at the mortuary.

(b) Government may intervene where mortal remains are not claimed within two days.

(c) Should the death rate appear to exceed the capacity of available space to keep mortal remains, the Government may intervene to facilitate mass burials.

(d) District and metropolitan municipalities should identify land that can be used for mass burial should a need arise.

(e) Municipalities should ensure that a mass burial is done in consideration of human dignity and necessary controls should be put in place to ensure that mortal remains can be identified.

(f) Machinery (for digging and closing of graves) can be used if deemed fit to prevent further spread of the virus and when hand tools are used during digging and closing the grave. The tools must be sanitised.

(g) People carrying the coffin must wear disposable hand gloves which must be disposed of properly.

Burial of Non COVID-19 mortal remains

81. (1) A mortuary staff member or an undertaker must not keep the mortal remains for more than 10 days from the date of death.

(2) Non COVID-19 mortal remains must be buried or cremated within 10 days from the date of death.

Appendix 3: *Extract from Department of Health. 2020. Circular on testing of all persons passing on at home or out of a health facility. 12 August.*

The Minister of Health in his media briefing held on the 5th August 2020 announced that "as part of improving the records of COVID-19 related deaths in response to reports on excess deaths, we now require that all the sudden deaths and those that occur at home must have specimens taken for COVID-19 before a death certificate is issued".

All persons who die at home must be tested for SARS Cov-2 by a Medical Doctor/ Clinician. The Medical Doctor/ Clinician that certifies the death and fills in the DHA Form 1663 form must also take the above-mentioned samples. Testing must be done before the human remain(s) are released to the funeral undertaker. The Medical Doctor/ Clinician must indicate on the DHA 1663 form that SARS Cov-2 samples have been taken. The sampling process should not interfere with prescribed time frames set for keeping human remains during the state of disaster period. If post-mortem testing is indicated, the clinician should always advise that the body must be managed as if it were COVID-19 positive.

The Department has taken several activities to assess whether the plateau that is observed in some provinces is due to reduced testing numbers or if indeed less people are becoming infected with Coronavirus.

It is critical that everyone dealing with death registration and confirmation assist the Department of Health to correctly record the cause of death by undertaking the testing as indicated above so that the country can have proper records.

NOTES

PRELIMS

1. Mda 1993 p. 10.

INTRODUCTION: COVID AND CUSTOM

1. Interview, Nelly Sharpley, 14/5/2020.
2. Bhongo, 29/10/2021.
3. Staunton, Swanepoel and Labuschaigne 2020; Francis 2020.
4. Staunton, Swanepoel and Labuschaigne 2020 p. 55.
5. See, for example, Friedman 2021.
6. See Giorgio Agamben 1998, 2004, 2020.
7. See Sotiris 2020; Corradetti and Pollicino 2021.
8. See De Waal 2020; Richards 2016.
9. See Silva and Higuera 2021.
10. Ibid; Ross 2011; see also Agamben 1998.
11. See Staunton, Swanepeol and Labuschaigne 2020 for further detail.
12. See Evans 2019 and Switzer 1993 for literature on this topic.
13. See De Waal 2020.
14. Ibid p. 10.
15. Ibid p. 12.
17. Foucault 1975.
18. Toscano 2020.
19. See Farmer 1996, 2020; Corradetti and Pollicino 2021.
20. De Waal 2020, 2021.
21. Staff writer, *Times*, 11/1/2021.
22. Giorgio Agamben 2003, 2020.
23. See Farmer 1996, 2003, 2020.
24. Bernault 2020.
25. Friedman 2020, 2021; see Francis 2020.

26. Ibid.
27. Ibid.
28. Bernault 2020.
29. Richards 2016.
30. De Waal 2021.
31. Ibid.
32. Richards 2016; Lipton 2020.
33. Paterson 2020; Dell and Paterson 2020.
34. Richards 2016; Niehaus 2018; Fairhead 2015; Leach 2020.
35. See Leach 2020; Tett 2021.
36. Scheper-Hughes 1993.
37. Fassin 2007; Niehaus 2018; Henderson 2012; Hosegood 2007, 2009; Camlin 2014; Nzioka 2002; Hunter 2010; Posel 2003.
38. Treatment Action Campaign 2013.
39. See Thornton 2008; also see Gelfand 2021.
40. Ibid.
41. Interview, Nelly Sharpley, 10/7/2020.
42. Wilson and Thompson 1969; Kanton and Kenny 1976; Lipton 1986.
43. See Beinart and Dubow 1995; Lipton 2007; Friedman 2015.
44. Wolpe 1972; Legassick 1974.
45. Mafeje 1981; Magubane 1973, 2007; Friedman 2015.
46. See Lee 2009; Bank, Posel and Wilson 2020; White 2010; Whyte 2013; Hickel 2015; Borges 2020.
47. Cohen 2020, Cohen and Sirkeci 2011; Cohen and Jonsson 2011; Awedeba and Hahn 2014; Collinson 2016; Moodie and Ndashe 1994; Bekker 2002.
48. Lee 2009; Posel 2003; Posel and Casale 2021; Hunter 2010; Du Toit and Neves 2014; Neves and Du Toit 2013.
49. See Posel and Cassale 2021.
50. Polanyi 1944; Gluckman 1970; Gudeman and Hann 2015; Gudeman 2008; Guyer 1993; Hann and Hart 2011; Healy-Clancy and Hickel 2014; Guyer 1993, 2018; Standing 2019; Kaneff and Endres 2021.
51. Polanyi 1944; Gluckman 1970; Hann 2014, 2018; Cash 2015; Gregory 2009; Hann and Hart 2011; Feffer 2017; Standing 2019; Kaneff and Endres 2021.
52. Also see Healy-Clancy and Hickel 2014; Ferguson 1992, 2013, 2015; Hann and Hart 2011; Shipton 2009; Fontein 2011; Jeske 2020.
53. See Visagie and Turok 2021.

1. HOMELANDS REMADE

1. Mbeki 1964; Laurence 1976; Southall 1982; Kepe and Ntsebeza 2011.
2. Hammond-Tooke 1963, 1975; Matoti and Ntsebeza 2020.
3. Carton and Morrell 2008; Mager 1998, 1999; Breckenridge 1990.
4. Peires 1987, 1989; Mostert 1992; Mda 2000.
5. Ibid.

6. Mostert 1992; Stapleton 1996, Wilson and Thompson 1969; Hamilton, Mbenga and Ross 2009.
7. Webster 1995; Lester 2001; Hamilton, Mbenga and Ross 2009; Braun 2014.
8. Switzer 1993; Braun 2014; Dubow 2006; Tropp 2006; also see Scott 1988; Evans 1997; Prices 2008 for social engineering and the colonial state.
9. Crais 2002, 2011; Beinart and Dubow 1995; Dubow 2006.
10. Crais 2011; Webster 1995.
11. Mostert 1992; Hamilton, Mbenga and Ross 2009; Wilson and Thompson 1969.
12. Redding 2020; Ross 2008.
13. Mayer 1971, 1980; Broster 1967, 1981.
14. Beinart 1980; Kepe and Ntsebeza 2011.
15. Reid 2020; Braun 2014.
16. Crais 2002; Beinart and Dubow 1995.
17. See especially Beinart 1982.
18. See Bundy 1988.
19. Switzer 1992; Wotshela 2020.
20. Crais 2011.
21. McAllister 2006; Hammond-Tooke 1963.
22. Geertz 1963; also see Hann and Hart 2011; Gudeman and Hann 2015.
23. Geertz 1960, 1983; White 1983.
24. Geertz 1969; Gudeman 2008.
25. McAllister 2006; Bourdieu 2000.
26. Wolpe 1972; Legasick 1974; Beinart 1980.
27. McAllister 2006; Bourdieu 2000.
28. Dietler, in McAllister 2006 pp. 56–65.
29. McAllister 2006 p. 16.
30. McAllister 2006 p. 26.
31. McAllister 2006; Kuckerts 1990; Hammond-Tooke 1963; Fay 2005.
32. Redding 2020 pp. 40–58.
33. Ibid.
34. Ibid.
35. Hunter 1936; Soga 1932.
36. Soga 1932; Reading 2020.
37. Carton and Morrel 2008, Mager 1999, 2002.
38. McAllister 2006 p. 154.
39. Carton and Morrell 2008.
40. Bank, Posel and Wilson 2020.
41. O'Connell 1980; Moodie and Ndatshe 1994.
42. Mager 2018.
43. Lodge 1984, 1986, 2011; Bank 2021a.
44. Crais 2002; Maaba 2004.
45. Maaba 2004; Lodge 1986.
46. Lodge 1984, 1986, 2011; Pieterse 2011.

47. Bank 2021b.
48. De Wet 2002; McAllister 1996; Beinart 2003.
49. McAllister 2001.
50. Mbeki 1964; Wiley 2001; Redding 2006; Pieterse 2011; Southall 1982.
51. Hammond-Tooke 1975; Kepe and Ntsebeza 2011; Lodge 1984, 1986.
52. See Mbeki 1964; Maaba 2004.
53. Ibid.
54. Sampson 1969; Broster 1967; Mayer 1971, 1980.
55. Ibid.
56. Ibid.
57. Bank 2015, 2020a, 2020b; Fay 2015.
58. Bank 2001, 2011; Bekker 2002.
59. Bank, Posel and Wilson 2020; Bekker 2002.
60. Visagie and Turok 2021.
61. Whiteside 2016.
62. Robins 2010; Hunter 2010.
63. Robins 2006; Steinberg 2009.
64. Interview, East London Health Committee, 20/10/2020.
65. Govere 2016; Steinberg 2009.
66. Lee 2011 pp. 235–247.
67. Ibid.
68. Jewekes and Morrell 2010; Hosegood et al. 2007.
69. Steinberg 2010.
70. Hosegood 2009; Camli 2014; Collinson 2010.
71. Mda 1995.
72. Bank 2010.
73. Case 2008.
74. Bähre 2011, 2019.
75. Dennie 2009; Ngubane 2004.
76. Bank 2015, 2020b.
77. Bank 2015; Fay 2015; Perry 2017.
78. See Beinart 2012 on the afterlife of homelands with special reference to the Transkei.

2. DEATH AND NAKED LIFE

1. See Bähre 2007; Leslie Bank's interviews with undertakers in high-density shack settlements in Cape Town revealed that, besides those who went home to the Eastern Cape, bodies were flown all over Africa for burial in 2018.
2. Ibid. In 2020, the British-based insurance company Sun Life estimated that South Africa was the fourth most expensive country in which to die after Japan, China and Germany as funeral costs exceeded 13% of the average annual wage, or cost R26,000 (or almost $2000) per funeral. However, given the very high unemployment level

in South Africa, the actual cost or investment for families in funerals relative to other costs is even higher; see Guy 2020.

3. The Disaster Management Act was passed in parliament in March 2020.
4. Feni 2020.
5. Ibid.
6. Ellis 2020.
7. Bank, Sharpley and Paterson 2020 p. 5.
8. Govere 2016; Steinberg 2008.
9. Gluckman 1937; Kuper 1982; Kuckertz 1990.
10. James 2009, 2014.
11. Hunter 1936 (1971) p. 227.
12. See Kuckertz 1990; McAllister 2006; Shipton 2009.
13. Hunter 1936 (1971) pp. 230–232.
14. Hunter 1936 (1971) p. 229.
15. Hunter 1936 (1971) p. 235.
16. Hunter 1936 (1971) p. 231.
17. Siphe Potelwa 2016 p. 10.
18. Interview, Phila Dyantyi 14/6/2020.
19. De Wet and Mgululwa 2020.
20. Ibid.
21. See Evans 2019 for a detailed account of forced removals in the Eastern Cape.
22. James 2009.
23. Stonington 2020; also see Lee 2011, 2012, 2013.
24. Steinberg 2008; McAllister 2006.
25. Lee and Vaughan 2008; Lee 2011, 2012; also see Gluckman 1937, 1970; Geschiere 2005; Evans-Pritchard 1949.
26. Stonington 2020.
27. Ibid pp. 50–64.
28. Lee 2011, 2013.
29. Block 2001; Dube 2001; Ballim 2013.
30. Bank, Posel and Wilson 2020; Lee 2009.
31. Bank 2015, 2020c.
32. Bank, Posel and Wilson 2020.
33. Case 2003 p. 34.
34. Naidu, in Potelwa 2016 pp. 50–52; Rand / £ exchange rate is 20:1.
35. Siphe Potelwa 2016 p. 86.
36. Smith 2004; Lee 2011.
37. Lee and Vaughan 2008.
38. Newell 2016; Hahn 2014.
39. Interview, Nelly Sharpley, 24/5/2020.
40. Interview, Dr Somododa Fikeni, 10/8/2020.
41. Interview, Nelly Sharpley, 24/5/2020.
42. Interview, Aneza Madini, 20/4/2020.

43. Feni, Fuzile and Piliso 2020.
44. BBC 2020.
45. Ibid.
46. Jubase and Ellis 2020.
47. WHO advisory April 2020.
48. Interview, Siyasanga, 10/6/2020.
49. Interview, Mandlakazi Tshunungwa, 24/6/2020.
50. Interview, Sanele Krishe, 27/8/2020.
51. Interview, Athi Phiwane, 23/5/2020.
52. Interview, Phelisa Nombile, 15/6/2020.
53. Sharpley 2021.
54. See Hickel 2016 for a detailed account of this process.
55. Interview, Sanele Krishe, Willowvale, 27/8/2020.
56. Interview, Balinda Mayosi, 24/6/2020
57. Interview, Vuyiswa Taleni, 2/7/2020.
58. Interview, Buleka Shumane, 30/6/2020.
59. Interview, Mandlakazi Tshunungwa, 10/7/2020.
60. Interview, Aneza Madini, 30/5/2020.
61. Interview, Puleng Morori, 21/5/2020.
62. Interview, Balindi Mayosi, 24/6/2020.
63. See Bank, Sharpley and Paterson 2020 pp. 21–25.

3. DISPOSABLE CITIZENS

1. Friedman 2020, 2021.
2. Ibid.
3. Ibid.
4. Ellis 2021a.
5. Ibid.
6. Bam 2021.
7. Farmer 2003, 2020.
8. Wylie 2001.
9. Marks 1994.
10. Ibid.
11. Hull 2017.
12. Marks 1994 p. 78.
13. See Bank and Qebeyi 2017.
14. Wylie 2002 pp. 130–45.
15. Wylie 2002 pp. 35–140.
16. Hull 2017 pp. 20–30.
17. Hull 2017; also see Jeske 2020; Hickel 2015.
18. Hull 2017.
19. Steinberg 2008; Govere 2016; Henderson 2012.

20. Ibid.
21. Treatment Action Campaign 2013.
22. Ibid.
23. Nkosi 2020.
24. Ibid.
25. Street 2014.
26. Ibid; also see Livingstone 2012.
27. Ellis 2021a.
28. Ibid.
29. Ibid.
30. Harding 2020.
31. See Harding 2020; Ellis 2020; Mnwana 2020.
32. Sizani 2020.
33. Nini 2020.
34. Bhongo and Nini 2020. The estimated death rate of two to three times the official rate was suggested by funeral parlour officials who suggested that many people had died at home and en route to hospital and had thus not been counted in the official figures.
35. Harding 2020.
36. Ibid.
37. Bhongo and Nini 2020.
38. Bhongo 2020.
39. Staff reporter 2020.
40. Ndebele 2020.
41. Ibid.
42. *Daily Maverick* Series on Health Worker Stories, October 2020.
43. Ibid; also see Kahn and Kelly 2001.
44. Ndebele 2020.
45. Mpulo 2020.
46. Ibid.
47. Mehlwana 2020.
48. Ibid.
49. Ibid.
50. Foster et al. 2020.
51. Jeranji 2020.
52. Ibid.
53. Ibid.
54. Ibid.
55. Ibid.
56. Interview, Nelly Sharpley, July 2020.
57. Ibid.
58. Ibid.
59. Interview, Athi Phiwani, 10/8/2020.
60. Ibid.

61. Ibid.
62. IInterview, Zipho Xego, 12/9/2020, with a 69-year-old cleric and religious leader in Lusikisiki.
63. Ibid.
64. Interview, Aneza Madini, 12/6/2020.

4. DIVIDED HOMESTEADS

1. Dandekar and Ghai 2020 p. 30; also see Khan and Arokkiaraj 2021 for overview.
2. See Bank 2020b for commentary on Covid-19 and reverse migration in South Africa.
3. Neves and Du Toit 2013; Du Toit and Neves 2014; Lee 2009.
4. See Bank, Posel and Wilson 2020.
5. Posel and Casale 2021 p. 6.
6. McAllister 2001.
7. Hebinck 2020.
8. White 2010.
9. Ibid.
10. See Hebinck 2020; Ngwane 2001, 2003.
11. Interview, Thabo, Engcobo, 23/9/2020.
12. Interview, Nelly Sharpley, July 2020.
13. Ngwane 2001, 2003.
14. Ngwane 2001, 2003; also see McAllister 2001.
15. Turok and Visagie 2021 p. 5.
16. Ibid.
17. Ibid.
18. Guyer 1993, 2018.
19. Ferguson 2013, 2015.
20. Hickel 2015.
21. Rice 2017.
22. Ibid.; see also Ferguson 2013.
23. Hickel 2016.
24. Rice 2017, 2020.
25. Hall and Posel 2017; Hall 2017.
26. Ibid.
27. Hall 2017; Bank 2020a, 2020b.
28. See Ntombana 2011; Ngxamngxa 1971; Vincent 2008; Jewkes and Morrell 2010.
29. Interview, Leslie Bank, 10/7/2020.
30. See the Acknowledgements for details.
31. In the latter half of 2020, President Ramaphosa frequently described GBV as a twin pandemic with Covid-19 in South Africa; also see Vincent 2008; Jewkes and Morrell 2010
32. See Bank 2020a, 2020b, 2020c for details.
33. See Dlamini 2021.

34. Geschiere 1990.
35. Ashworth 2005.
36. Niehaus 2001, 2012.
37. Mavhungu 2000.
38. Mchunu 2020.
39. See Lodge 1983, 2011; Maaba 2004.
40. Petrus 2009, 2011; also see Comaroff and Comaroff 2004.
41. Stadler 2014.
42. Comaroff and Comaroff 2004.
43. Niehaus 2001, 2011.
44. Crais 2002.
45. Staff reporter 2020.
46. Fuzile 2020.
47. Staff reporter 2019.

5. GATEKEEPERS

1. This chapter makes use of quotes from interviews which are too numerous to individually cite. The body of fieldwork described in the Acknowledgements is the basis for this chapter and the views expressed below.
2. Trengove 2017.
3. See Stadler 2021; Niehaus 2019.
4. Richards 2016; Leach 2019; Tett 2019; Farmer 2020.
5. See Farmer 2020 for the struggle between MSF and the WHO over this issue.
6. Ibid.
7. Tett 2021 pp. 68–69.
8. Asala 2020.
9. Southall 1980.

6. EXHUMING BODIES

1. See Tett 2021; Fairhead 2015; Leach 2018; Richards 2016.
2. Southall 2018 p. 23.
3. Butler 2008.
4. Interview, Mandlakazi Tshunungwa, 4/6/2020.
5. Interview, Eastern Cape House of Traditional Leaders, September 2021.
6. See Niehaus 2019; Stadler 2010.
7. See Bank, Sharpley and Paterson 2020 pp. 80–85.
8. Ellis, Jubase and Dlamini 2021; Ellis 2022.
9. Ibid.
10. The province was constantly in the media. In early 2022, the South African government reported by that: "By 7 February 2022 16,361 people in the province had been confirmed dead of Covid-19-related complications in just under two years.

The Medical Research Council estimated another 50,257 excess deaths due to natural causes in May 2020. Their estimation of 764 per 100,000 of the population puts the Eastern Cape death rate among the highest in the world and by far the highest in South Africa"; in Ellis 2022.

11. Interview, Eastern Cape House of Traditional Leaders, September 2020.
12. He described GBV as a parallel pandemic in South Africa, see Dlamini 2021.
13. Ibid.
14. Interview, Vuyiswa Taleni, 8/5/2020.
15. Interview, Phila Dyantyi, 10/4/2021.
16. Ibid.
17. Interview, Eastern Cape House of Traditional Leaders, September 2020.
18. Ibid.
19. Quoted in BBC 2020.
20. Ibid.
21. Interview, Phelisa Ellen Nombila, 15/5/2020.
22. Ibid.
23. Interview, Willowvale, May 2020.
24. Interview, Sanele Krishe, 17/6/2021.
25. Interview, Zipho Xego, 21/8/2020.
26. Interview, Zipho Xego, 5/10/2021.
27. *Daily Dispatch*, 20 October 2020.
28. Ibid.
29. Ellis 2021.
30. Ibid.
31. Harding 2020; Ellis, Jubase and Dlamini 2021; Ellis 2022.
32. Ellis 2022 reports that: "Hospital figures at the height of the (second) wave at the end of November and December showed that 26% of patients admitted to hospitals in the province had died, with 75% of deaths occurring in the public sector. But then December came and the province recorded more than 600 deaths, including the demise of 137 health workers, in the first two weeks." The same report states that: "By 7 February 2022 16,361 people in the province had been confirmed dead of Covid-19-related complications in just under two years. The Medical Research Council estimated another 50,257 excess deaths due to natural causes in May 2020. Their estimation of 764 per 100,000 of the population puts the Eastern Cape death rate among the highest in the world and by far the highest in South Africa."
33. Interview, Nelly Sharpley, 10/11/2020.
34. Ngwane 2003.
35. Interview, Singa Siyasanga, 15/1/2021.
36. Ibid.
37. Bank and Kenyon 2020 p. 274.
38. Ibid p. 276.
39. *Daily Dispatch*, 14 November 2020.
40. Ibid.

41. Interview, Puleng Morori, 9/12/2020.
42. Case recorded in *City Press*, December 2020.
43. Interview, Singa Siyasanga, 19/1/2021.
44. Interview, Athi Phiwane, 28/1/2021.
45. Interview, Siyasanga Fayini, 8/1/2021.
46. See Sharpley 2020.

CONCLUSION: POST-COVID RESET

1. Piot 2012; Judis 2016; Cas Mudde and Kaltwasser 2017; Lendvai 2018; Eatwell and Goodwin 2018; Krastev and Holmes 2019; Kaneff and Endres 2021.
2. Ibid.
3. Robins 2006, 2010; Lee 2009; Barchiesi 2011; Francis 2020; Southall 2020; Bank, Posel and Wilson 2020.
4. Ibid.
5. Ibid.
6. On the response to liberalism see especially Eatwell and Goodwin 2018; Krastev and Holmes 2019.
7. Ibid.
8. See Judis 2016; Mudde and Kaltwasser 2017 on populism.
9. Hickel 2015.
10. Ibid p. 45.
11. Marinovich 2016.
12. See Bank 2019.
13. Piot 2012; Reed 2020; Dlamini 2009; Bank and Mabhena 2011; Worby and Ally 2013; Paret 2018.
14. Bank and Mabhena 2011; Reed 2020.
15. Sizane 2020.
16. *Daily Maverick* news coverage of the election, 4/11/2021.
17. Gudeman and Hann 2015; Gudeman 2008; Gregory 2009; Guyer 1993; Hann and Hart 2011.
18. Ibid.
19. See especially Szelenyi 1988 on the Hungarian petty bourgeoisie.
20. Gudeman and Hann 2015; Gregory 2009; see also Kaneff and Endres 2021.
21. Ibid.
22. Ibid.
23. Krastev and Holmes 2019.
24. Gudeman and Hann 2015 p. 14–15.
25. See Heibinck 2020.
26. James 2015, 2017.
27. Interview, Zipho Xego, 10/10/2021.
28. Ibid.
29. Potelwa 2016 p. 54.
30. Moore 1994; Fraser 1995, 2016.

31. See Stadler 2021.
32. Ellis 2022.
33. Ibid.
34. Stadler 2021.

BIBLIOGRAPHY

Agamben, Giorgio. 1998. *Homo Sacer: Sovereign Power and Bare Life*. Stanford, CA: Stanford University Press.
———. 2004. *State of Exception*. Chicago, IL: Chicago University Press.
———. 2020. "L'invenzione di un'epidemia." Quodlibet. (translation).
Ainslie, Andrew. 2014. "Harnessing the ancestors: Mutuality, uncertainty and ritual practice in the Eastern Cape Province, South Africa." *Africa* 84 (4): 530–552.
Ashworth, Adam. 2005. *Witchcraft Violence and Democracy in South Africa*. Chicago, IL: Chicago University Press.
Assala, Kizzi. 2020. "Covid-19 upsets South African burial traditions." *Afrinews*, 10 August.
Awedoba, Albert and Hans Peter Hahn. 2014. "Wealth, consumption and migration in West African society." *Anthropos* 109: 45–55.
Ballim, Faeeza. 2013. "Burial in debt: high costs live on." *Mail and Guardian*, 28 March.
Bam, Bonile. 2021. "New Covid-19 grants, old Sassa problems." *Mail and Guardian*, 23 March.
Bank, Leslie. 2001. "Living together, moving apart: Home-made agendas, identity politics and urban-rural linkages in the Eastern Cape, South Africa." *Journal of Contemporary African Studies* 19 (1): 129–147.
———. 2011. *Home Spaces, Street Styles: Contesting Power and Identity in a South African City*. London: Pluto Press.
———. 2015. "City slums, rural homesteads: Migrant culture, displaced urbanism and the citizenship of the serviced house." *Journal of Southern African (Special Issue: Homelands as Frontiers: Apartheid's Loose Ends)* 41 (5): 1067–1081.
———. 2019. "Migrancy, war and belonging: The cultural politics of

African nationalism at Marikana." *Transformation: Critical Perspectives on South Africa* 100: 1–27.

————. 2020a. "Marikana revisited: Migrant culture, ethnicity and African nationalism in South Africa." In Leslie Bank, Dorrit Posel and Francis Wilson, eds. *Migrant Labour after Apartheid: The Inside Story*. Cape Town: HSRC Press.

————. 2020b. "Covid-19 reveals migration links in South Africa's Human Economy." *Daily Maverick*, 17 May. https://www.dailymaverick. co.za/article/2020-05-17-covid-19-reveals-migration-links-in-south-africas-human-economy/

————. 2020c. "Rural retreat: Allowing people to return home during lockdown." *Mail and Guardian*, 30 April. https://mg.co.za/article/2020-04-30-rural-retreat-allowing-people-to-return-home-during-lockdown-could-turn-a-tide/

————. 2021a. "Ground zero: Deep-seated colonial prejudice fuelled the pandemic in the rural Eastern Cape." *Daily Maverick*, 24 February. https://www.dailymaverick.co.za/article/2021-02-24-ground-zero-deep-seated-colonial-era-prejudice-fuelled-the-pandemic-in-rural-eastern-cape/

————. 2021b. "Covid and culture: How socially 'loose' South Africa can 'tighten' up for the third wave." *Daily Maverick*, 12 March. https://www.dailymaverick.co.za/article/2021-03-12-culture-and-covid-19-can-socially-loose-sa-tighten-up-its-response-before-the-third-wave/

Bank, Leslie and Michael Kenyon. 2020. "Cattle after migrant labour: Emerging markets and changing regimes of value." In Leslie Bank, Dorrit Posel and Francis Wilson, eds. *Migrant Labour after Apartheid: The Inside Story*. Cape Town: HSRC Press.

Bank, Leslie and Clifford Mabhena. 2012. "Bring back Kaiser Matanzima? Communal land, traditional leaders and the politics of nostalgia." In John Daniel, Prishani Naidoo, Devan Pillay and Roger Southall, eds. *New South African Review 2: New Paths, Old Compromises*. Johannesburg: Wits Press.

Bank, Leslie and Aneza Madini. 2021. "The politics of cultural defiance: Exhumations and rural reburials in Covid times." *Daily Maverick*, 7 February. https://www.dailymaverick.co.za/article/2021-02007-the-politics-of-cultural-defiance-exhumations-and-rural-reburials-in-covid-times/

Bank, Leslie and Mxolisi Qebeyi. 2017. *Imonti Modern: Picturing the Life and Times of a South African Location*. Cape Town: HSRC Press.

Bank, Leslie, Nelly Sharpley and Mark Paterson. 2020. *Closing the Gate: Death, Dignity and Distress in the Rural Eastern Cape in the Time of Covid*. Report for the Eastern Cape Socio-Economic Consultative Council (ECSECC), September.

BIBLIOGRAPHY

Bähre, Erik. 2007. *Violence and Money: Financial Self-help Groups in a South African Township*. Leiden: Brill.

————. 2020. *Ironies of Solidarity: Insurance and the Financialisation of Kinship in South Africa*. London: Zed Books.

BBC. 2020. "How 'secret burials' in South Africa could help tackle Covid-19." BBC, 11 May. https://www.bbc.com/news/world-africa-52571862

————. 2021 "Most African countries have incomplete death registration systems." BBC, 10 February.

Beinart, William. 1982. *The Political Economy of Pondoland, 1860–1930*. Cambridge: Cambridge University Press.

————. 2003. *The Rise of Conservation in South Africa: Settlers, Livestock, and the Environment 1770–1950*. Oxford: Oxford University Press.

————. 1987. "Conflict in Qumbu: rural consciousness, ethnicity and violence in the colonial Transkei." In William Beinart and Colin Bundy, eds. *Hidden Struggles in Rural South Africa*. Berkeley: University of California Press.

————. 2012. "Beyond homelands: Some ideas about the history of African rural areas in South Africa." *South African Historical Journal* 64 (1): 5–21.

Beinart, William and Saul Dubow. 1995. *Segregation and Apartheid in Twentieth-century South Africa*. London and New York: Routledge.

Bekker, S. 2002. *Migration Study in the Western Cape 2001*. Report for the Provincial Government of the Western Cape, Cape Town.

Bernault, Florence. 2020. "Some lessons from the history of epidemics in Africa." *Debating Ideas*. African Arguments, 5 June.

Bhongo, Jacob. 2020. "56 staff at one Eastern Cape hospital test positive for Covid-19." *Eastern Cape Herald*, 22 June.

Bhongo, Jacob and Asanda Nini. 2020. "Buckle up for Covid storm, warns Eastern Cape Premier." *Daily Dispatch*, 29 July.

Block, Robin. 2001. "Passing fancy: The lavish funerals South Africa favour come under threat." *Wall Street Journal*, 8 August.

Borges, Antonadia. 2020. "Land as home in South Africa: The living and the dead in ritual conversation." *Agrarian South: Journal of Political Economy* 9 (3): 275–300.

Bourdieu, Pierre. 2000. *Principles of an Economic Anthropology*. Translated by Chris Turner from Pierre Bourdieu, *Les Structures Sociales de l'économie*. Cambridge: Polity.

Braun, Lindsay. 2014. *Colonial Survey and Native Landscapes in Rural South Africa, 1850–1913*. Leiden: Brill.

Breckenridge, Keith. 1990. "Migrancy, crime and faction fighting: The role of the Isitshozi in the development of ethnic organisations in the compounds." *Journal of Southern African Studies* 16 (1): 55–78.

BIBLIOGRAPHY

Broster, Joan. 1967. *Red Blanket Valley.* Johannesburg: Hugh Keartland.
––––––. 1981. *Amagqirha: Religion, Magic and Medicine in Transkei.* Goodwood, South Africa: Via Afrika Ltd.
Bundy, Colin. 1988. *The Rise and Fall of the South African Peasantry.* 2nd ed. Cape Town: David Philip.
Butler, Anthony. 2008. *Cyril Ramaphosa.* Johannesburg: Jacana.
Butler, Judith. 1990. *Gender Trouble: Feminism and the Subversion of Identity.* New York: Routledge.
Camlin, Carol, Rachel Snow and Victoria Hosegood. 2014. "Gendered patterns of migration in rural South Africa." *Population, Space and Place* 20: 528–551.
Carton, Benedict. 2000. *Blood from Your Children: The Colonial Origins of Generational Conflict in South Africa.* Charlottesville: University of Virginia Press.
Carton, Benedict and Robert Morrell. 2012. "Zulu masculinities, warrior culture and stick fighting: reassessing male violence and virtue in South Africa." *Journal of Southern African Studies* 38 (1): 31–53.
Case, Anne, Anu Garrib, Alicia Menedez and Analia Olgiata. 2013. "Paying the piper: The high cost of funeral in South Africa." *Economic Development and Cultural Change* 63 (1): 1–18.
Cash, Jennifer. 2015. "Economy as ritual: The problems of paying in wine." In Stephen Gudeman and Chris Hann, eds. *Economy and Ritual: Studies of Postsocialist Transformations.* New York: Berghahn Books.
Chauke, Paballo. 2020. "Thief in the night: Covid took my Mom." *Mail and Guardian*, 19 January.
Cohen, Jeffery and Sirkeci, Ibrahim. 2016. "Migration and insecurity: Rethinking mobility in a neo-liberal age." In James Carrier, ed. *After the Crisis: Anthropological Thought, Neoliberalism and Its Aftermath.* London: Routledge.
Cohen, Robin and Gunvor Jonsson, eds. 2011. *Migration and Culture.* Cheltenham: Edward Elgar.
Collinson, Mark. 2010. "Striving against adversity: The dynamics of migration, health and poverty in rural South Africa." *Global Health Action* 3 (1): 1–13.
Comaroff, Jean and John L. Comaroff. 1993. *Modernity and Its Malcontents: Ritual and Power in Postcolonial Africa.* Chicago. IL: University of Chicago Press.
––––––. 2004. "Policing culture, cultural policing: Law and social order in postcolonial South Africa." *Law Society Inquiry* 29 (3): 513–533.
Corradetti, Claudio and Oreste Pollicino. 2021. "The war against Covid-19: State of exception, state of siege, or emergency (constitutional) pow-

ers?: The Italian case in comparative perspective." *German Law Journal* 22 (6): 1060–1071.

Crais, Clifton. 2002. *The Politics of Evil: Magic, State Power, and the Political Imagination in South Africa*. New York: Cambridge University Press.

———. 2011. *Poverty, War, and Violence in South Africa*. New York: Cambridge University Press.

Daily Dispatch. 2020. "ICU beds full at Port Elizabeth public hospitals as Covid-19 cases surge again." *Dispatch*, 11 November.

Dandekar, Ajay and Rahul Ghai. 2020. "Migration and reverse migration in the age of Covid-19." *Economic and Political Weekly* 55 (19): 1–9.

Dennie, Garrey. 2009. "The standard of dying: Race, indigence, and the disposal of the dead body in Johannesburg, 1886–1960." *African Studies* 68 (3): 310–330.

De Waal, Alex. 2020a. *New Pandemics, Old Politics: Two Hundred Years of War on Disease and Its Alternatives*. Cambridge: Polity Press.

———. 2020b. "New pathogen, old politics." *Boston Review*, April.

De Wet, Chris. 1995. *Moving Together, Living Apart: Betterment Planning and Villagisation in a South African Homeland*. Johannesburg: Wits Press.

De Wet, Chris and Erik Mgujulwa. 2020. "Innovative reworkings of ancestor ritual as a response to forced villagisation: An Eastern Cape example." *Anthropology Southern Africa* 43 (4): 246–258.

Dlamini, Jacob. 2009. *Native Nostalgia*. Johannesburg: Jacana.

Dlamini, Judy. 2021. "Gender-based violence, twin pandemic to COVID-19." *Critical Sociology* 47 (4–5): 583–590.

Dube, Vuyani. 2001. "Funeral become glamour, bereaved pressurised." *Pretoria News Weekend*, 27 October.

Dubow, Saul. 2006. *A Commonwealth of Knowledge: Science, Sensibility, and White South Africa, 1820–2000*. Oxford: Oxford University Press.

———. 2015. "Racial irredentism, ethnogenesis, and white supremacy in high-apartheid South Africa." *Kronos: Southern African Histories* 41 (1): 236–264.

Du Toit, Andre and David Neves. 2014. "The government of poverty and the arts of survival: Mobile and recombinant strategies at the margins of the South African economy." *Journal of Peasant Studies* 41 (5): 20–43.

Eatwell, Roger and Matthew Goodwin. 2018. *National Populism: The Revolt Against Liberal Democracy*. Milton Keynes: Pelican.

Ellis, Estelle. 2020a. "Gender based violence is South Africa's second pandemic, says Ramaphosa." *Daily Maverick*, 18 June.

———. 2020b. "Zweli Mhize: We are riding into a decimating and devastating storm." *Daily Maverick*, 24 June.

———. 2021a. "Death and dying in the Eastern Cape continued: What do you do when losing hope is not an option?" *Daily Maverick*, 15 July.

————. 2021b. "Eastern Cape government admits it has severe specialist shortages at hospitals." *Daily Maverick*, 29 March.

————. 2021c. "Toxic mess: Debt crisis leads to medical waste pile up at Eastern Cape hospitals." *Daily Maverick*, 8 March.

————. 2022. "A losing battle: Why mortality rates in one province rocketed during the Covid-19 second wave." *Daily Maverick*, 14 February.

Ellis, Estelle, Hoseya Jubase and Lonwabo Damani. 2021. "Swift and cruel: Investigation into high Eastern Cape Covid-19 death rate shows many died in casualty units." *Daily Maverick* (A Province at Breaking Point Series), 24 March.

Ellis, Estelle, Luvuyo Mehlwana and Zukiswa Pikoli. 2021. "Survival of the fittest: Battle for help at Eastern Cape clinics." *Daily Maverick* (A Province at Breaking Point Series), 26 March.

Evans, Ivan. 1997. *Bureaucracy and Race: Native Administration in South Africa*. Berkeley: University of California Press.

Evans, Laura. 2019. *Survival in the "Dumping Grounds": A Social History of Apartheid Relocation*. Leiden: Brill.

Evans-Pritchard, Edward. 1949. "Burial and mortuary rites of the Nuer". *African Affairs* 49 (190): 56–63.

Fairhead, James. 2016. "Understanding social resistance to Ebola response in the forest region of the republic of Guinea: An anthropological Perspective." *African Studies Review* 59: 7–31.

Farmer, Paul. 1996. "On suffering and structural violence: A view from below." *Daedalus* 125 (1): 261–293.

————. 2003. *The Pathologies of Power: Health Human Rights and the New War on the Poor*. Berkeley: University of California Press.

————. 2020. *Fever Feuds and Diamonds: Ebola and the Ravages of History*. New York: Farrar, Straus and Giroux.

Fassin, Didier. 2007. *When Bodies Remember: Experiences and Politics of AIDS in South Africa*. Berkeley: University of California Press.

Fay, Derick. 2005. "Kinship and access to land in the Eastern Cape: Implications for land tenure reform." *Social Dynamics* 31 (1): 182–207.

————. 2015. "'Keeping land for their children': Generation, migration and land in South Africa's Transkei." *Journal of Southern African Studies* (*Special Issue: Homelands as Frontiers: Apartheid's Loose Ends*) 41 (5): 1083–1097.

Feffer, John. 2017. *Aftershock: A Journey into Eastern Europe's Broken Dreams*. London: Zed Books.

Feni, Lulameli. 2020. "Many Eastern Cape rural areas ignoring lockdown restrictions." *Daily Dispatch*, 6 April.

Feni, Lulamile, Bongani Fuzile and Mfundo Piliso. 2020. "Shock as forty test positive for Covid-19 in tiny Port St Johns village." *Daily Dispatch*, 25 April.

Ferguson, James. 1992. "The cultural topography of wealth: Commodity paths and the structure of property in rural Lesotho." *American Anthropologist* 94 (1): 55–74.

———. 2013. "Declarations of dependence: Labour, personhood, and welfare in Southern Africa." *Journal of the Royal Anthropological Institute* 19 (2): 223–42.

———. 2015. *Give a Man a Fish: Reflections on the New Politics of Redistribution*. Durham, NC: Duke Press.

Fontein, Joost. 2011. "Graves, ruins, and belonging: Towards an anthropology of proximity." *Journal of the Royal Anthropological Institute* 17 (4): 706–727.

Foster, Isabel, Phumeza Tisile, Ingrid Schoeman and Ruvandi Nathavitharana. 2020. "Under-paid and under-protected: The case for supporting Community Health Workers." *Spotlight*, 28 September.

Foucault, Michel. 1975. *Abnormal: Lectures at the Collège de France, 1974–1975*. Translated by Graham Burchell. London: Verso.

Francis, David, I. Valodia and Eddie Webster. 2020. "Politics, policy, and inequality in South Africa under COVID-19." *Agrarian South* 9 (3): 342–355.

Fraser, Nancy. 1995. "From redistribution to recognition? Dilemmas for justice in a 'post-socialist' age." *New Left Review*, 212.

———. 2016. "Contradictions of capitalism and care." *New Left* Review, 100.

Friedman, Steven. 2015. *Race, Class and Power: Harold Wolpe and the Radical Critique of Apartheid*. Pietermaritzburg: University of KwaZulu-Natal Press.

———. 2020. "How South Africa's leaders unwittingly sabotaged Covid-19 effort." *Daily Maverick*, 19 July.

———. 2021. "No cure for South Africa's colonised medical minds." *Daily Maverick*, 18 January.

Fuzile, Bongani. 2020. "Witchcraft and gender based violence in Senqu." *Daily Dispatch*, 10 August.

Geschiere, Peter. 2005. "Funerals and belonging: Different patterns in southern Cameroon." *African Studies Review* 48 (2): 45–64.

Gluckman, Max. 1937. "Mortuary customs and the belief in survival after death amongst the south-eastern Bantu." *Bantu Studies* 11: 117–36.

———. 1970. *Custom and Conflict in Africa*. Oxford: Basil Blackwell.

Govere, Fredrick. 2016. *Pills, Partners and Politics: Governing the HIV-AIDS Pandemic in the Eastern Cape*. PhD thesis, University of Fort Hare.

Gregory, Chris. 2009. "Whatever happened to householding?" In Chris

BIBLIOGRAPHY

Hann and Hart Keith, eds. *Market and Society: The Great Transformation Revisited*. Cambridge: Cambridge University Press.

Guy, Duncan. 2020. "The high cost of dying in South Africa." *IOL News*, 22 August.

Gudeman, Stephen. 2008. *Economy's Tensions: The Dialectics of Community and the Market*. New York: Berghahn Books.

Gudeman, Stephen and Chris Hann. 2015. "Introduction: Ritual, economy and the institutions of the base." In Stephen Gudeman and Chris Hann, eds. *Economy and Ritual: Studies of Postsocialist Transformations*. New York: Berghahn Books.

Guyer, Jane. 1993. "Wealth in people and self-realisation in Equatorial Africa." *Man* 28 (2): 243–265.

———. 2018. "Pauper, percentile, precarity: Analytics from poverty studies in Africa." *Journal of African History* 59 (3): 437–448.

Hahn, Hans Peter. 2015. "Consumption in Africa." In Daniel Cook and Michael Ryan, eds. *The Wiley Blackwell Encyclopaedia of Consumption and Consumer Studies*. London: John Wiley & Sons.

Hall, Katherine. 2017. *Children's Spatial Mobility and Household Transitions: A Study of Child Mobility and Care Arrangements in the Context of Maternal Migration*. PhD thesis, University of the Witwatersrand.

Hamilton, Carolyn, Bernard Mbenga and Robert Ross, eds. 2009. *The Cambridge History of South Africa*. Vol. 1. Cambridge: Cambridge University Press.

Hammond-Tooke, W. David. 1963. "Kinship, locality and association: Hospitality groups among the Cape Nguni." *Ethnology* 2 (3): 302–319.

———. 1975. *Command or Consensus: The Development of Transkeian Local Government*. Cape Town: David Philip.

Hann, Chris. 2014. "The economistic fallacy and forms of integration under and after socialism." *Economy and Society* 43 (4): 626–649.

———. 2018. "Ritual and economy: From mutual embedding to festivalisation in provincial Hungary." *Lietuvos Etnologij* 18 (27): 9–34.

Hann, Chris and Keith Hart. 2011. *Economic Anthropology: History, Ethnography and Critique*. Cambridge: Polity Press.

Harding, Andrew. 2020. "Coronavirus in South Africa: Inside Port Elizabeth's 'hospital of horrors'." BBC, 15 July.

Hebinck, Paul. 2020. "Migrancy and the differentiated agrarian landscapes: Land-use, farming and the reproduction of the homestead in the Eastern Cape in Bank." In Leslie Bank, Dorrit Posel and Francis Wilson, eds. *Migrant Labour after Apartheid*. Cape Town: HSRC Press.

Henderson, Patricia C., 2012. *A Kinship of Bones: AIDS, Intimacy and Care in Rural KwaZulu-Natal*, Scottsville: University of KwaZulu-Natal Press.

Hickel, Jason. 2011. "On the politics of home." In M. Healy-Clancy and

J. Hickel, eds. *Ekhaya: The Politics of Home in KwaZulu-Natal*. Pietermaritzburg: University of KwaZulu-Natal Press.

————. 2015. *Democracy as Death: The Moral Order of Anti-liberal Politics in South Africa*. Berkeley: University of California Press.

Hosegood, Victoria. 2009. "The demographic impact of HIV and AIDS across the family and household life cycle: Implications for efforts to strengthen families in sub-Saharan Africa." *AIDS Care* 21 (1): 13–21.

Hosegood, Victoria, Eleanor Preston-Whyte, Joanna Busza, Moitse Sindile and Ian Timaeus. 2007. "Revealing the full extent of household experiences of HIV and AIDS in rural South Africa." *Social Science and Medicine* 65: 1249–1259.

Hull, Elizabeth. 2017. *Contingent Citizens: Professional Aspiration in a South African Hospital*. London: Bloomsbury Academic.

Hunter, Mark. 2002. "The materiality of everyday sex: Thinking beyond 'prostitution'." *African Studies* 61 (1): 99–120.

————. 2006. "Fathers without *amandla*: Zulu-speaking men and fatherhood." In Linda Richter and Robert Morrell, eds. *Baba: Men and Fatherhood in South Africa*. Pretoria: HSRC Press.

————. 2010. *Love in the Time of AIDS: Inequality, Gender, and Rights in South Africa*. Bloomington: Indiana University Press.

Hunter, Monica. 1936. *Reaction to Conquest: Effects of Contact with European on the Pondo of South Africa*. Cape Town: Oxford University Press.

James, Deborah. 2009. "Burial sites, informal rights and lost kingdoms: Contesting land claims in Mapumulanga." *Africa* 79 (2): 228–251.

————. 2014. *Money from Nothing: Indebtedness and Aspiration in South Africa*. Stanford, CA: Stanford University Press.

Jeranji, Tiyese. 2020. "Innovating and adapting at the rural Zithulele Hospital during Covid-19." *Daily Maverick*, 2 October.

Jeske, Christine. 2020. "People refusing to be wealth: What happens when South African workers are denied access to 'belonging in'." *Economic Anthropology* 7 (2): 253–266.

Jewkes, Rachel and Robert Morrell. 2010. "Gender and sexuality: Emerging perspectives from the heterosexual epidemic in South Africa and implications for HIV risk and prevention." *Journal of the International AIDS Society* 13 (1): 6–17.

Jubase, Husaya and Estelle Ellis. 2020. "Funerals suspended in parts of province as Covid-19 infections rise." *Daily Maverick*, 28 April. https:// www. dailymaverick.co.za/article/2020-04-28-funerals-suspended-in-parts-of-province-as-covid-19-infections-rise/

Judis, John. 2016. *The Populist Explosion: How the Great Recession Transformed American and European Politics*. New York: Columbia Global Reports.

Kahn, Mark S. and Kevin J. Kelly. 2001. "Cultural tensions in psychiatric nursing: Managing the interface between Western mental health care and Xhosa traditional healing in South Africa." *Transcultural Psychiatry* 38 (1): 35–50.

Kaneff, Deema and Kirsten W. Endres, eds. 2021. *Explorations in Economic Anthropology: Key Issues and Critical Reflections*. Oxford: Berghahn Books.

Kantor, Brian and Henry Kenny. 1976. "The poverty of neo-Marxism: The case of South Africa." *Journal of South African Studies* 3 (1): 20–40.

Kepe, Thembela and Lungusile Ntsebeza, eds. 2011. *Rural Resistance in South Africa: The Mpondo Revolts after Fifty Years*. Leiden: Brill.

Khan, Asma and H. Arokkiaraj. 2021. "Challenges of reverse migration in India: A comparative study of internal and international migrant workers in the Post-Covid economy." *Comparative Migrant Studies*, 9, 49.

Krastev, Ivan and Stephen Holmes. 2019. *The Light that Failed: A Reckoning*. Milton Keynes: Penguin Books.

Kuckertz, H. 1990. *Creating Order: The Image of the Homestead in Mpondo Social Life*. Johannesburg: Wits University Press.

Kuper, Adam. 1982. *Wives for Cattle: Bridewealth and Marriage in Southern Africa*. London: Routledge and Kegan Paul.

Laurence, Patrick. 1976. *The Transkei: South Africa's Politics of Partition*. Johannesburg: Ravan Press.

Leach, Melissa. 2015. "The Ebola crisis and post-2015 development." *Journal of International Development* 27 (6): 816–834.

Lee, Rebekah. 2009. *African Women and Apartheid: Migration and Settlement in Urban South Africa*. London: I. B. Tauris.

———. 2011. "Death on the move: Funerals, entrepreneurs and the rural-urban nexus in South Africa." *Africa* 81 (2): 226–247.

———. 2013. "Funeral frenzy: Mourner, entrepreneurs and the price of death in Africa." *Huffington Post*, 28 May.

Lee, Rebekah and Megan Vaughan. 2008. "Death and dying in the history of Africa since 1800." *Journal of African History* 49 (3): 341–359.

Leggassick, Martin. 1974. "South Africa: Capital accumulation and violence". *Economy and Society* 1 (1): 5–35.

Lendvai, Paul. 2018. *Orbán: Hungary's Strongman*. Oxford: Oxford University Press.

Lester, Alan. 2001. *Imperial Networks: Creating Identities in Nineteenth Century South Africa*. London: Routledge.

Liebenberg, Alida. 1997. "Dealing with relations of inequality: Married women in a Transkei village." *African Studies* 56 (2): 349–373.

Lipton, Jonah. 2020. "What Ebola taught me about Coronavirus: panic will get us nowhere." *The Guardian*, 11 March.

Lipton, Merle. 1986. *Capitalism and Apartheid*. London: Wildwood Press.

BIBLIOGRAPHY

————. 2007. *Liberals, Marxists and Nationalists: Competing Interpretations of South African History*. New York: Palgrave Macmillan.

Livingston, Julie. 2012. *Improvising Medicine: An Oncology Ward in an Emerging Cancer Epidemic*. Durham, NC: Duke University Press.

Lodge, Tom. 1984. *Black Politics in South Africa since 1945*. Johannesburg: Ravan Press.

————. 1986. "The Poqo insurrection, 1961–1968." In John Lonsdale, ed. *Resistance and Ideology in Settler Societies*. Johannesburg: Ravan Press.

————. 2011. *Sharpeville: An Apartheid Massacre and Its Consequences*. Oxford: Oxford University Press.

Maaba, Brown Bavusile. 2004. "The PAC's war against the state, 1960–1963." In South African Democracy Education Trust, ed. *The Road to Democracy in South Africa 1 (1960–1970)*. Cape Town: Zebra Press.

Mafeje, Archie. 1981. "On the articulation of modes of production: Review article." *Journal of Southern African Studies*. 8 (1): 123–138.

Mager, Anne. 1998. "Youth organisations and the construction of masculine identities in the Ciskei and Transkei, 1945–60." *Journal of Southern African Studies* 24 (4): 653–668.

————. 1999. *Gender and the Making of a South African Bantustan: A Social History of the Ciskei, 1945–59*. Portsmouth, NH: Heinemann.

Mager, Anne and Phiko Velelo. 2018. *The House of Tshatshu: Power, Politics and Chiefs North West of the Great Kei River, c.1818–2018*. Cape Town: UCT Press.

Magubane, Bernard. 1973. "The 'Xhosa' in town, revisited urban social anthropology: A failure of method and theory." *American Anthropologist* 75 (5): 1701–1715.

————. 2007. "Whose memory, whose history? The illusion of the liberal and radical historical debates." In Hans Erik Stolten, ed. *History Making and Present Day Politics: The Meaning of Collective Memory in South Africa*. Uppsala: Nordic Africa Institute.

Makhulu, Anne-Maria. 2015. *Making Freedom: Apartheid, Squatter Politics, and the Struggle for Home*. Durham, NC: Duke University Press.

Marinovich, Greg. 2017. *Murder at a Small Koppie: The Real Story of the Marikana Massacre*. Cape Town: Penguin.

Marks, Shula. 1994. *Divided Sisterhood: Race, Class and Gender in the South African Nursing Profession*. Johannesburg: Wits University Press.

Matoti, Sukude and Lungisile Ntsebeza. 2004. "Rural resistance in Mpondoland and Thembuland, 1960–1963." In South African Democracy Education Trust, ed. *The Road to Democracy in South Africa*. Cape Town: Zebra Press.

Mavhungu, Khaukanani N. 2000. "Heroes, villains and the state in South Africa's witchcraft zone." *African Anthropologist* 7 (1): 114–129.

BIBLIOGRAPHY

Mayer, Philip. 1971. "'Traditional' manhood initiation in an industrial city: The African view." In E. J. De Jager, ed. *Man: Anthropological Essays Presented to O.F Raum*: 7–18. Cape Town: Struik Publishers.

—————. 1980. "The origin and decline of two rural resistance ideologies." In Philip Mayer, ed. *Black Villagers in an Industrial Society*. Oxford and Cape Town: Oxford University Press.

Mayer, Philip and Iona Mayer. 1970. "Socialization by peers: The youth organization of the red Xhosa." In Philip Mayer, ed. *Socialization: The Approach from Social Anthropology*. London: Tavistock Publications.

—————. 1971. *Townsmen or Tribesmen: Conservatism and the Process of Urbaniza tion in a South African City*. Second edition. Cape Town: Oxford University Press.

Mbeki, Govan. 1964. *South Africa: The Peasants' Revolt*. Harmondsworth: Penguin.

McAllister, Patrick. 2001. *Building the Homestead: Agriculture, Labour and Beer in South Africa's Transkei*. Ashgate: African Studies Centre, Leiden.

—————. 2005. "Xhosa co-operative agricultural work groups: Economic hindrance or development opportunity?" *Social Dynamics* 31 (1): 208–234.

—————. 2006. *Xhosa Beer Drinking Rituals: Power, Practice and Performance in the South African Rural Periphery*. Durham, NC: Carolina Academic Press.

Mchunu, Mxolisi. 2020. *Violence and Solace: The Natal Civil War in Late Apartheid South Africa*. Pietermaritzburg: University of KwaZulu-Natal Press.

Mda, Zakes. 1993. *When People Play People: Development Communication through Theatre*. Johannesburg: Wits Press.

—————. 1995. *Ways of Dying*. New York: Picador.

—————. 2000. *In the Heart of Redness*. New York: Picador.

Mehlwana, Luvuyo. 2020. "Dire conditions at Mthatha General and Nessie Knight hospitals." *Spotlight*, 29 September.

Mhlanga, David. 2004. "Think of dignity and don't get into debt." *The Sowetan*, 22 July.

Mnwana, Sonwabile. 2020. "The Eastern Cape is in a Covid-19 crisis—time to mobilise our unemployed youth." *Daily Maverick*, 9 July.

Moodie, T. Dunbar and Vivienne Ndatshe. 1994. *Going for Gold: Men, Mines, and Migration*. Berkeley: University of California Press.

Moore, Donald. S. 2005. *Suffering for Territory: Race, Place and Power in Zimbabwe*. London: Duke University Press.

Moore, Henrietta. 1994. "Households and gender in a South African Bantustan: A comment." *African Studies* 53 (1): 137–142.

Morrell, Robert. 1998. "Of boys and men: Masculinity and gender in southern African studies." *Journal of Southern African Studies* 24 (4): 605–630.

BIBLIOGRAPHY

Mostert, Noel. 1992. *Frontiers: The Epic of South Africa's Creation and the Tragedy of the Xhosa People*. New York: Knopf.

Mpulo, Nontsikelelo. 2020. "The Eastern Cape health crisis is nothing new." *Spotlight*, 2 July.

Mudde, Cas and Christobal Kaltwasser. 2017. Populism: *A Very Short History*. Oxford: Oxford University Press.

Murray, Colin. 1981. *Families Divided: The Impact of Migrant Labour in Lesotho*. Cambridge: Cambridge University Press.

Ndebele, Nomatter and Thom Pierce. 2020. "Eastern Cape doctor: We know that whenever we treat sick people, we risk getting infections." *Daily Maverick*, 2 October.

Neves, David and Andre Du Toit. 2013. "Rural livelihoods in South Africa: Complexity, vulnerability and differentiation." *Journal of Agrarian Change* 13 (1): 93–115.

Newell, Sasha. 2016. *The Modernity Bluff: Crime, Consumption and Citizenship in Côte d'Ivoire*. Chicago, IL: University of Chicago Press.

Ngubane, Harriette. 2004. "Traditional practices on burial systems with special reference to the Zulu people of South Africa." *Indilinga: African Journal of Indigenous Knowledge Systems* 3 (2): 171–177.

Ngwane, Zolani. 2001. "'Real men reawaken their fathers' homesteads, the educated leave them in ruins': The politics of domestic reproduction in post-Apartheid rural South Africa." *Journal of Religion in Africa* 31 (4): 402–426.

———. 2003. "Christmas time and the struggles for the households in the countryside: Rethinking the cultural geography of migrant labour in South Africa." *Journal of Southern African Studies* 29 (3): 681–699.

Ngxamngxa, A. N. N. 1971. "The function of circumcision amongst the Xhosa-speaking tribes in historical perspective." In E. J. De Jager, ed. *Man: Anthropological Essays Presented to O.F Raum*. Cape Town: Struik Publishers.

Niehaus, Isak. 2001. *Witchcraft, Power and Politics: Exploring the Occult in the South African Lowveld*. London: Pluto Press.

———. 2007. "Death before dying: Understanding AIDS stigma in the South Africa Lowveld." *Journal of Southern African Studies* 33 (4): 845–860.

———. 2012. *Witchcraft and a Life in the New South Africa*. Cambridge: Cambridge University Press.

———. 2018. *AIDS in the Shadow of Biomedicine: Inside South Africa's Epidemic*. London: Zed Books.

———. 2019. "Seeing through dreams: On the efficacy of anti-retroviral drugs in the South African Lowveld." *Journal of Southern African Studies* 45 (1): 197–213.

Nini, Asanda. 2020. "Virus shuts down East Cape police stations." *Dispatch Live*, 19 May. https://www.dispatchlive.co.za/news/2020-05-19-virus-shuts-down-eastern-cape-police-stations/

Nkosi, Makeni. 2011. "The funerals that cost families dear." BBC, 26 November.

Ntombana, Luyuvo. 2011. *An Investigation into the Role of Xhosa Male Initiation in Moral Regeneration.* PhD thesis, Nelson Mandela Metropolitan University.

Ntsebeza, Lungisile. 2005/2006. *Democracy Compromised: Chiefs and the Politics of Land in South Africa.* Cape Town and Leiden: HRSC Press and Brill.

Nzioka, Charles. 2002. "The social meanings of death from HIV/AIDS: An African interpretative view." *Culture, Health and Sexuality* 2 (1): 1–14.

Paret, Marrcel. 2018. "Critical nostalgias in democratic South Africa." *Sociological Quarterly* 59 (4): 678–696.

Paterson, Mark and Leslie Bank. 2021. "Fear of the body: How the government got it wrong on Covid-19 burials." *Daily Maverick*, February. https://www.dailymaverick.co.za/article/2021-02-01-fear-of-the-dead-how-the-government-got-it-wrong-on-covid-19-burials/

Peires, Jeff. B. 1982. *The House of Phalo: A History of the Xhosa People in the Days of Their Independence.* Los Angles: University of California Press.

———. 1987. "The central beliefs of the Xhosa cattle-killing." *Journal of African History* 28 (1): 43–63.

———. 1989. *The Dead Will Arise: Nongqawuse and the Great Xhosa Cattle-Killing Movement.* Johannesburg: Ravan Press.

Perry, Adam. 2017. *Building the Homestead in Willowvale.* PhD thesis, University of Fort Hare.

Pieterse, Jimmy. 2011. "Reading and writing the Mpondo revolts." In Thembela Kepe and Lungisile Ntsebeza, eds. *Rural Resistance in South Africa: The Mpondo Revolts after Fifty Years.* Leiden: Brill.

Pigg, Stacy Lee. 1992. "Inventing social categories through place: Social representations and development in Nepal." *Comparative Studies in Society and History* 34 (3): 491–513.

Petrus, Theodor. 2009. *An Anthropological Study of Witchcraft-related crime in the Eastern Cape and Its Implications for Law Enforcement Policy and Practice.* PhD thesis, Nelson Mandela University.

———. 2011. "Defining witchcraft-related crime in the Eastern Cape Province of South Africa." *International Journal of Sociology and Anthropology* 3 (1): 1–8.

Polanyi, Karl. 1944. *The Great Transformation: The Political and Economic Origins of our Times.* Boston, MA: Beacon.

BIBLIOGRAPHY

Posel, Dorrit. 2003. "Have migration patterns in post-apartheid South Africa changed?" Paper presented at the conference on African Migration and Urbanisation in Comparative Perspective. Johannesburg. Available at: http://www. pum.princeton.edu/pumconference/papers.html

Posel, Dorrit and Daniela Casale. 2021. "Moving during times of crisis: Migration, living arrangements and COVID-19 in South Africa." *Scientific African* (13).

Potelwa, Siphe. 2016. *The Visual Narrative Relating to Social Performance of the Xhosa People during Burial*. Master's thesis in Visual Art, University of South Africa.

Price, Richard. 2008. *Making Empire: Colonial Encounters and the Creation of Imperial Rule in Nineteenth-century Africa*. Cambridge: Cambridge University Press.

Redding, Sean. 2006. *Sorcery and Sovereignty: Taxation, Power and Rebellion in South Africa, 1880–1963*. Athens: University of Ohio Press.

———. forthcoming. *Gender, Violence and the Reconstitution of Tradition in South Africa*. Charlottesville, VA: University of Virginia Press.

Reed, Amber. 2020. *Nostalgia after Apartheid: Disillusionment, Youth, and Democracy in South Africa*. Notre Dame, IN: University of Notre Dame Press.

Reid, Darren. 2020. "Dispossession and the legal mentality in nineteenth century South Africa." *Settler Colonial Studies* 11 (1): 69–85.

Rice, Kate. 2014. "*Ukuthwala* in rural South Africa: Abduction marriage as a site of negotiation about gender, rights and generational authority among the Xhosa." *Journal of Southern African Studies* 40 (2): 381–400.

Rice, Kathleen. 2017. "Rights and responsibilities in rural South Africa: Implications for gender, generation, and personhood." *Journal of the Royal Anthropological Institute* 23 (41): 28–41.

Riesman, Paul. 1986. "The person and the life cycle in African social life and thought." *African Studies Review* 29 (2): 71–138.

Robins, S. L. 2008. *From Revolution to Rights in South Africa: Social Movements, NGOs and Popular Politics After Apartheid*. Scottsville: University of KwaZulu-Natal Press.

Robins, Steven. 2006. "From 'rights' to 'ritual': AIDS activism in South Africa." *American Anthropologist* 108 (2): 312–323.

Ross, Fiona. 2011. *Raw Life, New Hope: Decency, Housing and Everyday Life in a Post-apartheid community*. Cape Town: University of Cape Town Press.

Sampson, H. F. 1969. *The White-Faced Huts: Witchcraft in the Transkei*. Johannesburg: Voortrekker.

Scorgie, Fiona. 2002. "Virginity testing and the politics of sexual responsibility: Implications for AIDS intervention." *African Studies* 61 (1): 55–75.

BIBLIOGRAPHY

Scott, James. 1988. *Seeing like a State: How Certain Schemes to Improve the Human Condition Have Failed*. New Haven, CT: Yale University Press.

Sizani, Mkhuseli. 2020. "PE clinic closes after nurse dies and 11 staff test positive for Covid-19." *Ground Up*, 12 May.

Sharpley, Nelly. 2021. "The buttons that hold together: *Umakoti* in the face of Covid-19." In Amanda Gouws and Olivia Ezeobi, eds. *COVID Diaries: Women's Experience of the COVID-19 Pandemic*. Cape Town: Imbali Academic Press.

Shipton, Parker. 2009. *Mortgaging the Ancestors: Ideologies of Attachment*. New Haven, CT: Yale University Press.

Silva, Guillermo and Christina Higuera. 2021. "Political theology and COVID-19: Agamben's critique of science as a new 'pandemic religion'." *Open Theology* 7 (1): 501–513.

Smith, Nicholas Rush. 2019. *Contradictions of Democracy: Vigilantism and Rights in Post-Apartheid South Africa*. Oxford: Oxford University Press.

Soga, John Henderson. 2013 [1932]. *The Ama-Xosa: Life and Customs*. Cambridge: Cambridge University Press.

Sotiris, Panagiotis. 2020. "Against Agamben: Is democratic biopolitics possible?" *Viewpoint Magazine*, 20 March.

———. 2020. "Democratic biopolitics revisited: A response to a critique." *Critical Legal Thinking* 25: 1–15.

Southall, Roger. 1982. *South Africa's Transkei: The Political Economy of an "Independent" Bantustan*. London: Heinemann.

———. 2020. *The New Black Middle Class in South Africa*. Oxford: James Currey.

Spiegel, Andrew. 1997. "Continuities, culture and the commonplace: Searching for a new ethnographic approach in South Africa." In P. McAllister, ed. *Culture and the Commonplace: Anthropological Essays in Honour of David Hammond-Tooke*. Johannesburg: Witwatersrand University Press.

———. 1995. "Migration, urbanization and domestic fluidity: Reviewing some South African examples." *African Anthropology* 2 (2): 90–113.

Stadler, Jonathan. 2003. "Rumour, gossip and blame: Implications for HIV/ AIDS prevention on the South African Lowveld." *AIDS Education and Prevention* 15 (4): 357–368.

———. 2021. *Public Secrets and Private Suffering in the South African AIDS Epidemic*. New York: Springer.

Staff reporter. 2019. "Witchcraft murders leave Mbizana residents living in fear." *SABC News*, 21 May.

———. 2020. "Three witches killed for being witches." *Opera News*, July. https://za.opera.news/za/en/crime/f985bb41c-c0a13f75924f-cc01558d44d

BIBLIOGRAPHY

Standing, Guy. 2019. *Plunder of the Commons: A Manifesto for Sharing Public Wealth*, Milton Keynes: Pelican.

Stapleton, Timothy. 1996. "The expansion of a pseudo-ethnicity on the Eastern Cape: Reconsidering the Fingo 'Exodus' of 1865." *International Journal of African Historical Studies* 29: 233–250.

Staunton, Ciara, Carmen Swanepoel and Melodie Labuschaigne. 2020. "Between a rock and a hard place: Covid-19 and South Africa's response." *Journal of Law and Bioscience* 7 (1): 50–72.

Steinberg, Jonny. 2008. *Three-letter Plague: A Young Man's Journey through a Great Epidemic*. New York: Vintage.

Street, Alice. 2014. *Biomedicine in an Unstable Place: Infrastructure and person-hood in a Papua New Guinean Hospital*. Durham, NC: Duke University Press.

Switzer, Les. 1993. *Power and Resistance in an African Society: The Ciskei Xhosa and the Making of South Africa*. Pietermaritzburg: University of Natal Press.

Szelenyi, Ivan. 1988. *Socialist Entrepreneurs: Embourgeoisement in Rural Hungary*. Cambridge: Polity.

Tett, Gillian. 2021. "Contagion: Why can't medicine stop pandemics?" In *Anthro-vision: How Anthropology Can Explain Business and Life*. London: Random House.

Thornton, Robert. J. 2008. *Unimagined Community: Sex, Networks and AIDS in Uganda and South Africa*. Berkeley: University of California Press.

Toscano, Alberto. 2020. "Beyond the Plague State." *Public Goods*, May.

Treatment Action Campaign (TAC). 2013. *Death and Dying in the Eastern Cape: An Investigation into the Collapse of a Health System*. Section 27 NSP Review.

Trengove, John. 2020. *Inxeba* (The Wound) Film/Documentary, South Africa.

Tropp, Jacob. 2006. *Natures of Colonial Change: Environmental Relations in the Making of the Transkei*. Athens, OH: Ohio University Press.

Vincent, Louise. 2008. "'Boys will be boys': Traditional Xhosa male cir-cumcision, HIV and sexual socialisation in contemporary South Africa." *Culture, Health and Sexuality* 10 (5): 431–446.

Visagie, Justine and Ivan Turok. 2020. "Rural-urban inequalities amplified by COVID-19: Evidence from South Africa." *Area Development and Policy* 6 (1): 1–20.

Webster, A. 1995. "Unmasking the Fingo: The war of 1835 revisited." In Carolyn Hamilton, ed. *The Mfecane Aftermath: Reconstructing Debates in Southern African History*. Johannesburg and Pietermaritzburg: Witwatersrand University Press.

White, Hylton. 2010. "Outside the dwelling of culture: Estrangement and

BIBLIOGRAPHY

difference in postcolonial Zululand." *Anthropological Quarterly* 83 (3): 497–518.

White, Benjamin. 1983. "Agricultural involution and its critics: Twenty years after." *Bulletin of Concerned Asian Scholars* 15 (2): 18–31.

Whyte, S. R. 2005. "Going home? Belonging and burial in the era of AIDS." *Africa* 75 (2): 154–174.

Whiteside, Alan. 2016. *HIV/AIDS: A Very Short History.* Oxford: Oxford University Press.

Wilson, Monica. 1981. "Xhosa marriage in historical perspective." In Eileen Jensen Krige and John L. Comaroff, eds. *Essays on African Marriage in Southern Africa.* Cape Town: Juta.

Wilson, Monica and Leonard Thompson, eds. 1969. *Oxford History of South Africa* (2 vols). New York: Oxford University Press.

Wolpe, H. 1972. "Capitalism and cheap labour power in South Africa: From segregation to apartheid." *Economy and Society* 1 (4): 425–456.

Worby, Eric and Shireen Ally. 2013. "The disappointment of nostalgia: Conceptualising cultures of memory in contemporary South Africa." *Social Dynamics* 39 (3): 457–480.

Wotshela, Luvuyo. 2018. *Capricious Patronage and Captive Land: The Politics of Resettlement and Change in South Africa's Eastern Cape, 1960–2005.* Pretoria: UNISA Press.

Wylie, Diane. 2001. *Starving on a Full Stomach: Hunger and the Triumph of Cultural Racism in Modern South Africa.* Charlottesville, VA: University of Virginia Press.

INDEX

Note: Page numbers in **Bold** indicate maps and followed by "*n*" refer to notes, "*f*" refers to figures